When
It
Hurts

Sabrina Shue, MD
with
Linda Morrison Spear

When It Hurts

Inside A Pain Management Doctor's Practice

Bink Books
Bedazzled Ink Publishing Company • Fairfield, California

paperback 978-1-949290-78-3

Cover Design
by

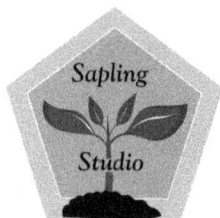

Sapling
Studio

Bink Books
a division of
Bedazzled Ink Publishing, LLC
Fairfield, California
http://www.bedazzledink.com

This book is dedicated to my family.

*My husband Min, whose love, encouragement, and support
allow me to pursue my dreams without reservations.*

*My children Seraphina, Vivianna, and Allydia, who are my biggest fans
and my sources of joy. Special thanks to Seraphina for
helping me edit the entire book.*

*My brother and sister in law, Danny and Jennifer,
whose friendship have given me strength and warmed my heart
especially during my most trying days as a new immigrant.*

*My mom and dad, who gave up everything to bring us to this country,
providing us with endless opportunities and possibilities.*

"Live as if you were to die tomorrow.
Learn as if you were to live forever!"
—*Mahatma Gandhi*

CONTENTS

PROLOGUE

"TO CURE SOMETIMES, TO RELIEVE OFTEN, AND TO COMFORT ALWAYS."

This quote well describes what we do as doctors in general. In chronic pain management, I think it can be more appropriately modified as, "To cure never, to relieve sometimes, and to comfort often."

It is important to explain to people exactly what doctors in the field of pain management do.

The questions I usually encounter include the following:

"You're an anesthesiologist? What's that? I've never heard about that job before."

"Why do you work in an office? Don't anesthesiologists only work in the operating room in hospitals?"

"Pain management? Your patients must be addicts."

Although the specialty of pain management has been around for a few decades, it is still relatively young. In contrast to the many well-known traditional medical specialties, like surgery or internal medicine, many patients have yet to fully explore and learn about what the field of pain management offers.

I am an interventional pain management doctor with a background in anesthesia. I mainly use interventional procedures, such as steroid injections and nerve blocks, which I will talk about later on in this book, to help chronic pain patients minimize their pain and suffering.

My patients are found in every age group, socio-economic level, and ethnicity. What they all have in common is their chronic pain.

No, my patients are not addicts. Or, at least, not that I am normally aware of, but it can be a tricky endeavor to identify them when they do appear.

While I was in medical school, I felt compelled to work with my hands to use various injections and minimally invasive procedures, to provide relief for my patients.

As a young physician, I believed that solid medical knowledge was the single most important cornerstone for any healthcare provider. If one cannot properly and accurately make the diagnosis, what good can the doctor do? I went through four years rigorous medical school training at the University of North Carolina at Chapel Hill, then completed a four-year residency in anesthesia at a Harvard affiliated hospital, and on to finish my training at a Columbia-affiliated interventional pain management fellowship. I was confident that I possessed the necessary fundamental knowledge base that would allow me to practice medicine in the best way I know how.

Before long, I realized that no education or medical training would prepare me enough for being a doctor in the real world.

The overall goal of chronic pain management is to reduce discomfort and to help patients return to daily living. While there are a variety of options available to treat chronic pain, it usually cannot be cured, only managed.

The longer I am in the field, that more I realize besides medical knowledge, it is equally, if not more important to offer a listening ear and comfort to patients, because often, that is the only thing I can do.

With no exceptions, we all, at one time or another, feel pain. Some of us handle it well; some of us wince at the slightest twinge. My patients' stories that follow will take you on a journey that my patients and I share and endear. I try to meet their needs with medical expertise, compassion, and hope; and I have learned so much from them in the process.

"I'm on the verge of a total breakdown. Sciatica. Taxes. Cars. Fleas, possibly. It's an absurd existence." — Jonathan Ames

"I Don't Want Surgery"

EACH MORNING FOR about three months, fifty-one-year-old Steve woke up with a wrenching pain in his low back and right hip, radiating down to the back of his right thigh and calf. This situation made it impossible for him to get started for work until he took some non-steroidal anti-inflammatory medication that helped him move around.

Within a half hour, his leg felt somewhat better—enough for him to shower, put on his clothes, and get ready to drive the one-hour trip to his office.

It didn't take Steve long to become annoyed each morning when he had to deal with the throbbing ache before he could begin his day.

He eventually contacted his primary care physician about the problem, who suggested that he come in to check out the issue.

Low back pain that spreads to hips and legs is one of the most common reasons that Americans visit their doctors. Each year, low back pain causes about 149 million lost days of work in the U.S. and costs $100 billion to $200 billion—mostly in lost wages and productivity.

The low back is an intricately created structure of interconnecting bones, joints, nerves, ligaments, and muscles all working together to provide support, strength, and flexibility to our bodies. However, this complex structure also leaves the low back susceptible to injury and discomfort. While about 85 percent of the low back pain resolves with minimal intervention, some people need more help and time.

The New York Times reported in February 2017, the American College of Physicians and the American Society released updated guidelines as follows:

"Given that most patients with acute or sub-acute low back pain improve over time, regardless of treatment, doctors and patients should select non-medication treatments, including topical heat, massage, acupuncture, or spinal manipulation.

For patients with chronic low back pain, non-medication treatments should be used first. These include exercises, multidisciplinary rehabilitation, mindfulness-based stress reduction, tai chi, yoga, motor control exercise, progressive relaxation, electromyography biofeedback, low-level laser therapy, cognitive behavioral therapy, or spinal manipulation.

Patients with chronic low back pain who do not get enough relief from the above-mentioned therapy, should consider pharmacological treatment with non-steroidal anti-inflammatory drugs as first-line therapy, tramadol, or duloxetine as second-line therapy along with muscle relaxants. Doctors should only consider opioids as an option in patients who do not respond to the other available treatments."

Steve's primary care doctor recommended that he take a course of ibuprofen, up to 800mg, three times a day with food, as needed; physical therapy three times a week and stretching exercises daily at home.

Six weeks passed, Steve was feeling about the same, without much improvement. His agony was making it miserable for him to tolerate his daily activities and work.

That was when the doctor suggested that Steve undergo a lumbar spine MRI and see a pain management specialist for further evaluations and treatments. On the suggestion of his doctor, he made an appointment with me.

After I introduced myself, I asked Steve to tell me where the pain was located.

"Didn't you review my MRI report," he practically shouted with obvious annoyance. "My problem is shown on the MRI report."

I was hardly surprised by Steve's question or his irritation. In fact, a good number of patients would show their annoyance when I ask them where it hurts, because they assume that the MRI results should have told me everything I need to know about their problem.

MRI has proven to be an extremely valuable tool in the assessment of normal and pathological spinal anatomy. However, like many other medical tests, MRI is not perfect. According to an article published in the *Journal of Orthopaedic Surgery and Research in* 2018, MRI was found to be 72 percent sensitive, 68 percent specific, and 70 percent accurate in determining the status of lumbar herniated discs.

This means that MRI may be inaccurate in assessing the status of lumbar disc herniation in 30 percent of cases. For many patients, the damaged parts that are seen on imaging studies do not always correlate with the source or the degree of distress.

The truth is that not everyone with a herniated disc on MRI has pain. Conversely, a clean MRI that shows no findings does not mean that the patient does not have low back pain. This study stresses the point that we should never treat solely based on an MRI and should always base treatment on the patient's symptoms and the results of a thorough physical examination.

Some doctors question if it is always wise for people to see their abnormalities on film because it can undermine their confidence that they can continue to lead a healthy, active life. Once they see that they are impaired, they may become a "backache patient" and that image can stay with them for the rest of their lives as a mental burden.

After listening to the whole story of Steve's problem and his complete medical history, I performed a physical examination. One of the tests I use is called the "straight leg raise test." Steve lay on his back with his legs fully stretched out and I slowly raised them, one at a time, and noted the elevation at which the pain began. Steve was yelping in agony when his right leg was raised, and he felt the same shooting pain down the back of his right thigh and calf. This test helped to confirm that something in his spine was pinching his nerve and creating the problem he experienced. Steve, otherwise, had normal muscle tone, strength, sensation, and reflexes.

"Now can you tell me what's really wrong with me," he asked with urgency. "My pain is getting worse in my hip and thigh, and I thought I might need a hip replacement. Why did my other doctor tell me my problem is in my back? My back hurts but that's not my main problem. And why does my pain feel different almost every day? It is like it has a mind of its own and it changes all the time."

Steve was so agitated that he looked like he might yell. It is difficult to deal with constant pain without becoming short tempered and snappish.

"I believe your pain emanates from an irritated or pinched nerve in the spine, Steve. People usually call this sciatica."

"I think that was what my primary doctor said too, but what does that mean?" he asked, as he cocked his head.

"Sciatica," I continued, "refers to pain that radiates along the buttocks and down each leg. Since sciatica is often felt in those areas, people usually mistake it for problems with their hips. No wonder you thought your hip joint was the dysfunctional problem.

"In fact, the sciatic nerves are formed by branches from spinal nerves coming down the lower back. Sciatica most commonly occurs when the spinal nerves, not the sciatic nerve itself, are being irritated when they exit areas of their origins. This symptom is really from a pinched spinal nerve, not from a problem with the sciatic nerve itself."

"Oh no," Steve replied with dread, "I have a pinched nerve. Now that's a real problem."

"Don't worry, Steve," I said, as I noticed his growing stress. "This is something we can treat and work on together."

The MRI film revealed that Steve had developed two lumbar disc herniations at the bottom of his spine at the level of L4/5, and L5/S1, impinging on his L5, and S1 spinal nerves on the right side. While any lumbar spinal nerve impingement can cause pain in the low back and buttock area, different spinal nerves control various territories in thighs and legs. That is why I always ask patients about the pattern of pain in their thighs and legs.

This Q and A with the patient helps the doctor determine which nerve root is really the reason for a patient's symptoms. Steve's L5, S1 nerve root problem explained why he had excruciating pain in his low back and the back of his right thigh and calf. If upper nerve roots are pinched, patients would feel shooting down to the outside, or the front of the thighs and legs.

I showed Steve where the yellow spinal nerves were in a lumbar spine model. "Imagine that your spinal nerves control everything in your legs, including all kinds of feelings and your strength. Depending on which nerve fibers are being irritated in any given moment, pain and discomfort can vary widely, from a mild ache to a sharp, burning sensation or excruciating pain. Sometimes it can feel like a jolt or an electric shock.

"Some people also have numbness, tingling or muscle weakness in the affected leg or foot. Others might have pain in one part of the leg and numbness in another part. Some patients describe it as itching, water running down their legs, hot irons poking, bugs crawling or a pins and needles sensation."

Steve's eyes widened at the thought of those symptoms. "Bugs crawling, and hot irons poking me, huh?"

I smiled and told him that herniated discs are the most common cause of narrowing of the spine and pinched nerves in young and middle-aged people.

"People like you, Steve. In older patients, pinched nerves are more likely to be from narrowing of the spine due to degenerative disc disease, arthritis, and spinal stenosis. No matter what the root cause of pinched nerves is, the collection of symptoms is similar, which is sciatica. "

We proceeded to talk more about the different treatment options for his condition.

"For pain associated with nerve impingement that is not responding to conservative treatments including NSAIDS, physical therapy, acupuncture, yoga, like in your case, we should consider the next step of treatment options," I explained.

"I don't want surgery!" he blurted out. "In fact, I won't have surgery." He peered at me. "Do you think I will need surgery?" His anxiety clearly overwhelmed him.

"Steve, calm down," I softly replied.

"There are only two reasons for which people would have surgery.. When a patient has weakness in the legs or feet, or starts to have bowel or bladder incontinence, it means the spinal nerve or the spinal cord is being severely compressed by the herniated disc. That patient has no choice but to have surgery. When a patient is in severe and uncontrollable pain, not responding to non-surgical treatments, he or she can choose to have surgery, although this patient still has a choice as long as there is no weakness or incontinence. You are not in either of these two situations now," I said to him with simplicity.

"Contrary to what most people believe, pain is not the worst sign for a lumbar disc problem, even though it can make people feel like it is the end of the world. Weakness is the deal breaker."

Steve released a huge sigh of relief that an operation would not be needed, especially since he had not as yet tried other less invasive treatment options.

"I suggest something different. I think that an injection of cortisone with lidocaine, delivered directly into the area of the slipped discs will help to reduce swelling and inflammation of the nerve roots. Once the nerve root is not being squeezed so tightly, your pain will lessen. After we do the injection, I also think that you should consider a round of physical therapy in which stretching exercises should improve your flexibility. You can also focus on core strengthening exercises. Your strong muscles can act as a natural belt around your waist to support your low back and prevent further injury."

"What is the difference between cortisone and steroid shots? Are these going to make me fat? Are they the same thing some athletes use to make themselves bulk up?" Steve asked.

"In this case, cortisone and steroid shots mean the same thing. Doctors and patients use these two terms interchangeably. Cortisone is a kind of steroid. It is short for corticosteroid, a human-made version of the hormone cortisol, which is different from the hormone-related steroid compounds that some athletes use. One needs worry about weight gain from high dose and long-term oral steroid use, not from a few injections."

"Some of my friends also had low back pain, but they got an epidural shot, whatever that is. How come I'm not getting that too?" Steve asked.

"Cortisone shots are injections that may help relieve pain and inflammation in a specific area of your body. They're most commonly injected into joints— such as your ankle, elbow, hip, knee, shoulder, spine, and wrist," I explained. "When this injection is given in the spine area, specifically in a location called the epidural space, to treat inflamed spinal nerves, the injection is also called epidural steroid injection. Therefore, a cortisone shot describes the medication used in the injection. An epidural injection describes the location of the injection. In fact, you will be getting a cortisone injection in the epidural space. You can call it either a cortisone shot or an epidural shot."

Steve nodded and shook my hand. Without a moment's hesitation, Steve chose to have the injection procedure.

Three days after the initial examination and assessment, Steve came back for the injection.

He lay on the operating table, face down, so that I could begin the procedure. An X-ray machine was used for me to determine the exact location for his injection. With every small incremental needle advancement, an X-ray picture was taken to ensure that the needle was aiming at the correct target.

Even though we try to treat a nerve root which does not show up on an X-ray, because the machine only sees bony structures; we have a particularly good idea where nerves would be in relationship to the bony landmarks.

Once I place the needles under X-ray guidance, I also use a small amount of contrast material to be certain that the needle is in the correct place. I want to be sure that the needle is not in a blood vessel and medication will flow only into the epidural space.

Within minutes, I placed the injections into the affected area and the procedure was complete. Steve was moved to recovery and felt considerably better, shortly thereafter.

The injection mixture contains a small amount of lidocaine, which is a numbing medicine, along with cortisone, which reduces the inflammation. When injected near irritated nerves in the spine, the lidocaine takes effect within minutes. That was why Steve already felt better while he was in the recovery room at my office.

Once the lidocaine wears off in a few hours, however, patients may feel their usual pain again, along with some new pain from the irritation from the needle or the procedure itself, which can last a couple to hours or even a day or two. Shortly thereafter, the cortisone in the mixture will start to take effect, reduce inflammation, and relieve the pain.

When the injections work, patients usually feel much better between two to five days. It's hard to predict what any individual person will experience, but the majority of people have at least partial relief for weeks to many months. Steroid injections do not reduce the lumbar disc herniation itself. The human body will try to do its own job to heal the injury. In the meantime, the medication can ease pain and discomfort and allow patients live their lives less affected by the problem.

Steve received a total of three treatments in the span of nine months. His pain became minimal, at worst, and he was one of the lucky ones. For one, his condition could be treated in an office setting and further treatment might not be necessary. But best of all, he could get back to coaching his son's softball team.

It's been more than a year since Steve received his injections and has not had a flair up. Physical therapy strengthened his core muscles, and he keeps up with his exercise routines on a regular basis.

For many other patients, however, pain from a herniated disc may linger and return. Steroid injections can be repeated but are usually limited to just a few a year because there's a chance these drugs might weaken the local soft tissue and bones. This problem isn't caused by the needle—it's a possible side effect of steroids, which include facial flushing, sleep and appetite disturbances, and moodiness. People with existing high blood pressure, and high blood sugar may see their numbers increase for a few days which usually return to baseline without intervention. The risk of side effects increases with the frequency of the number of steroid injections that the person receives.

For my patients who need epidural steroid injections on a regular basis, I always encourage them to wait as long as possible. After each treatment, I advise them to be active and do their core strengthening exercises daily.

I particularly worry about the effect of long-term cortisone use on my elderly female patients. Their bone density is at risk since most of them already have osteopenia or even osteoporosis. Cortisone is known to put patients at higher danger of further bone loss. However, if a patient is bed bound because of pain and leading a sedentary lifestyle, they are at risk of bone loss as well, along with higher risk of developing other medical problems and general health status decline. If steroid injections can allow patients to become more active, walk more and exercise more, the bone building effect of a healthful lifestyle will counteract the negative effects of steroids on bones.

I have had elderly patients riddled with pain from spine disease, begging me to give them more and more cortisone injections. When I tried to tell them about the harm due to overuse of cortisone, they sometimes cry. One of my older patients flatly said, "What is the use of my good bones down the years if I don't even want to live my life right now because of my terrible pain? Don't I also have a right to decide what to do with my own body?"

To treat or not to treat, the best answer only lies in an individual's specific needs and goals. Effective communication with patients to help them understand the pros, cons, and alternatives to each treatment is the best way to make these decisions together as a team.

My Perfect Patients

WHEN I FIRST hung my shingle as a pain management specialist, I did not give much thought as to why my patients would come to see me. Isn't that obvious? If a doctor is caring, compassionate, and technically skillful at what he or she does, the doctor will naturally be in high demand. Patients would be willing to drive long distances, get through heavy traffic and hassles, trek over mountains, and paddle across oceans, just to see this doctor.

When two brothers, Tim and Jack, showed up at my office, they had driven at least a hundred miles, round trip, to consult with me about their pain.

"Wow," I thought, "It must be that word has spread about me. Somebody must have told them that I am a good doctor."

I was getting a little excited. I could not help it. A hundred miles!

Tim and Jack, according to themselves, had been treated by a local doctor near them with methadone for their chronic low back pain and other work-related injuries. They had tried several types of pain management injections, physical therapy, non-narcotic medications—all without relief. Their doctor finally was able to keep their pain stable with a small amount of the methadone.

However, their doctor recently retired, and their primary care physician was not comfortable with prescribing methadone. They needed to find a new pain management physician to take over their care.

Methadone is part of a category of opioids that was created by German doctors during World War II. When it arrived in the United States, it was used to treat people in extreme pain. Most people have heard of methadone for its treatment of addiction to heroin, cocaine, or other opioids. A methadone maintenance program can quell the urge and prevent withdrawal symptoms. It is also widely used for management of chronic pain because it works a lot like morphine or OxyContin and is often taken as a tablet, just like any other pill.

As an interventional pain management specialist, I prefer to use non-medication methods for chronic pain control. However, I also realize that like anything in medicine, no specific method works for everyone. Some patients do need medication therapy. Our pain management training taught us that, if a patient was stable on opioids, not showing signs of misuse, abuse, or the need for escalating opioid dosage over time, then it would be okay to prescribe if the patient was under constant close monitoring.

During the initial visit, in addition to gathering their medical histories, physical examinations, and imaging studies and reports, I asked the Tim and Jack to leave a urine sample for toxicology analysis. I do this because I never give out any pain medications on the first visit. I need to do my homework first before I take them in as my patients.

After I finished seeing all patients that day, I called their primary care physician to verify that the brothers did not have any history of substance abuse, misuse, or any medication diversion. I then called their pharmacy to verify that there had been only one physician, their pain management doctor, who gave them the methadone; and methadone was the only opioid they had received.

I also called the previous pain management physician who had already closed his practice and was unreachable. However, the information from the primary care doctor and the pharmacy was clean and satisfactory. For Tim and Jack, my homework results did not raise any red flags regarding improper opioid prescription use.

I did not realize homework would continue after I graduated from decades of schooling, let alone I never liked homework. After a full day of patient care, the phone calls, the chasing after doctors and pharmacies sometimes made me forget what I went to medical school for in the first place. I never envisioned that in order to practice medicine, I needed to become a detective and a call center clerk out of necessity.

No one knows better than a physician or pharmacist that opioids are powerful and can be deadly. I had to protect patients and my practice by not letting opioids fall into the wrong hands. I had no choice but to do all my homework, for all my patients.

Two weeks later, Tim and Jack came for their follow-up appointments. We reviewed their toxicology screening results, which showed that all they had been taking, in terms of controlled substances, was the methadone. Otherwise, there was no illicit component in the urine sample. There were no street drugs, or other prescription medication that they could have borrowed or purchased from friends.

They passed.

We discussed the risk of taking long-term opioids, potential overdoses, and addiction problems. I also went over other non-narcotic options with them in detail. Finally, I had each of the brothers sign a narcotic contract.

This contract is a treatment agreement signed by the patient and the doctor that sets out the expectations for a patient using these high-risk medications. The use of a narcotic contract allows for the documentation of understanding between both parties. Such contract can improve communication between doctors and patients. Common contract elements include:

- Informing the patient of the risk of opioid tolerance and physiologic dependence
- Requiring that only one doctor prescribes, and one pharmacy dispenses the drug
- Stating that lost or stolen prescriptions will not be replaced
- Prohibiting dose or frequency increases by the patient
- Use of prescription drug monitoring programs
- Assessments of compliance, such as random pill counts and urine drug screens in the prescriber's office
- Agreement on the fact that violation of the contract would result in discharge of the patient

Tim and Jack agreed to the contract, and they signed them in front of me.

They continued to come for their monthly appointments for their refills of methadone and would bring their pill bottles for me to count their numbers of pills to ensure they were using the medication exactly as I had prescribed.

From time to time, I would ask for urine samples for a random toxicology analysis. They always passed. The urine toxicology results were undoubtedly clean every time.

Tim and Jack were always on time for medication refills. They never complained that their pain was worse, or they needed more medication.

The brothers were tall, burly men. However, they were always subdued, polite, and mild mannered when they were at my office. They complied with every of one of my requests with a smile. If I had any choice, patients like Tim and Jack would be the perfect ones to have as long-term patients. They were stable medically; no behavioral trouble at all.

Perfect.

"Not all weapons are guns or blades. The most dangerous are subtle, hidden." — Andrea Bremer

Risky Business

ABOUT ONE YEAR passed by since Tim and Jack became my patients. Things were going as usual, until one day, Phoebe, a regular patient of mine came to see me for a medication renewal. Phoebe had been with me for about two years. She was also on low dose methadone for her chronic knee pain. Phoebe had abused heroin in her youth. Through dirty needle use, she contracted a dreadful infection that almost killed her.

The infection lingered in her right knee, despite long-term intravenous antibiotic treatment. As a result, she required multiple knee surgeries to debride the infection which ate through her cartilage and knee joint.

Fortunately, she survived it all, but was left with a right knee that was badly deformed. Thus, she was relegated to crutches for the rest of her life.

"Well, as terrible as it was," she told me repeatedly, "I am grateful that I had the infection and got that sick. Otherwise, I probably would have died a long time ago from using heroin and cocaine. That hospitalization made me come clean. I have been sober for more than ten years now, and I'm stable on my methadone which helps my pain. It's not perfect, but I don't want anything more than that."

I was always grateful to hear these words from Phoebe. Over the years, Phoebe made no waves. All the ways in which we monitored, treated, and tested her, had shown clean results, just like the brothers, Tim and Jack.

This particular day, Phoebe leaned forward as soon as I closed the door in the consultation room. She looked from side to side and behind me, as if making sure nobody was following me, then drew me closer and said, "Dr. Shue, I saw two old acquaintances outside in your waiting room. Tim and Jack used to go to the same high school as my older brother. What a shock."

I looked at the schedule. The two brothers were supposed to be here a little later that day, however, they were almost always early for their appointments, because they said they did not want to be late, due to traffic or other potential tie-ups.

"Really, what a coincidence," I said no more because I worked to keep all patients' care and information confidential. Phoebe looked at me with slight hesitation in her eyes, but dropped the topic on Tim and Jack.

Two months later, Phoebe returned for another follow up visit. After the usual medical issues were discussed, Phoebe whispered, "I've thought about this for a long time but decided that I need to tell you something." She sidled up close to me. "You have got to promise that you are not going to tell anyone that I told you this. Otherwise, I'll get into big trouble."

"What is on your mind, Phoebe?" I was concerned.

"Those two brothers, Tim and Jack. I think I told you they are my brother's friends. My brother still spends time together with them." She paused. "They are selling methadone on the street. I assumed that it was the methadone they got from you if that's what you prescribe for them. I thought that you would want to know. Please, please don't tell anyone I told you this. They are bad people, and they would get me in big trouble, if you understand what I mean."

I stood still and felt a jolt of surprise go through my body.

I did not realize methadone had much value on the street. From Phoebe, I learned that methadone apparently had become a popular street drug because it was significantly less expensive than other opioids, which were also sold on the street.

I could not believe what I was hearing about my two "good" patients. I pretended to be calm as I thanked her for her concern and the information. I also promised that I would keep her identity confidential.

Phoebe walked out of my office with a trace of anxiety on her face and fear in her eyes.

It was a dilemma I had to face, head on. First of all, who should I trust? Tim, Jack, or Phoebe? Was Phoebe telling me the truth? What would she gain if she were making this story up? How and where could I get evidence on the alleged illicit drug sales and medication diversion?

If there was a deviation from the contract, it would be a breach of the relationship I had with Tim and Jack, and I would have to discharge them. Could I discharge them if I did not have any concrete evidence? After all, I could not possibly catch them red-handed if they sold their methadone on the street. What kind of burden of proof did I need to discharge a patient?

And why did I even have to worry about all this? Wasn't my job that of a physician, not a detective?

After much deliberation and some sleepless nights, I decided to discharge Tim and Jack. I couldn't take any chances with their behavior. Although they acted perfectly and sailed through all my monitoring efforts, it would not be difficult for these experienced people to beat the system. I had more trust in Phoebe, especially I did not see anything she could gain from telling on her brother's friends.

Now, what did I need to do to let Tim and Jack go?

It is no easy task for a physician to release a patient. If it is not done correctly, a physician can be accused of abandoning a patient—or worse. Again, I had to do my homework on how to release them.

According to the rules of medical treatment, to terminate a doctor and patient relationship, the patient should be formally dismissed with a written notice stating that he or she must find another healthcare practitioner.

If the discharge process cannot be done face to face, a written notice must be mailed to the patient by regular, as well as certified mail, return receipt requested.

I needed to keep copies of the letters to both patients, along with the original certified mail receipts, and the original certified mail return receipts, in their medical records. In the discharge letters, I assured them that I would provide alternative options for their medical care. I also had to provide a thirty-day supply of methadone for each, so that they would not go into withdrawal in the process of finding another pain management physician.

The day came when I had to confront Tim and Jack with the discharge letters. The usually polite and soft-spoken men became infuriated and ugly as they dealt with my disclosure.

In a fit of anger, one of them turned his back to me as he walked out the door and shouted, "Watch it! We'll be back."

He stomped out and slammed my office door, as his brother followed quickly behind him. One of my staff asked, "What did he mean? Is he going to come back with a gun?" I felt a chill going through my body, from head to toe.

What did he mean? Really? What did he mean?

I had my staff members watch the entrance of the building and had a phone in hand to call 911 immediately if they should return. I then surveyed my office. Now there was nowhere to hide or run. There would be nothing we could do to defend ourselves, other than wait for help to arrive.

To our immense relief, Tim or Jack did not return that day. Yet, our office remained open, and patients came and went every weekday thereafter. We knew the brothers could have come back at any time to harass us. And if so, what could we have done?

Over the next few months, one of the brothers would repeatedly call after office hours and leave messages on my voice mail screaming, "Give me my methadone, bitch!" His voice chilled me to the bone.

I decided to call the police and register a complaint with the local precinct in order to ensure immediate response from them, should we be placed in danger.

After a while, the messages finally stopped, but my worry did not end. I knew very well that there could be another Tim or Jack in the future, who would appear initially as a perfect patient, but later turn out to be a monster.

I learned my lesson. I no longer confront patients with difficult issues while alone in the consultation room. If I need to deliver unwanted news, such as a discharge or refusal to prescribe opioids, I am accompanied by another staff member. When I anticipate unruly patient behaviors, I ask my strongest staff to wait outside the door and break in if I scream for help.

Being a physician can be a risky business. Who knew? I surely didn't know. When I was young, I had amiable relationships with my own doctors. I just made the assumption that it would all be polite and pleasant in patient and doctor interactions.

After my experience with Tim and Jack, when I see people come to me from far away, I would pay special attention. One can never know why a patient goes through extra hassle to see a pain management physician. Is it because the patient is too notorious for a local physician to take him or her on for treatment? Or is it because the wait time at other physicians' offices is really too long? Or, are the local doctors truly all as terrible as they describe? Or, some friends and family in fact said all these good words about me? When I try to pick out the problematic patients. It's like a cat and mouse game but only much harder. Even with all the appropriate questioning, calls to pharmacies and physicians, investigations, narcotic contracts, urine toxicology and behavior monitoring, I can still be fooled.

If you search the Internet, you will find a plethora of websites and online forums which would inform people how to beat a pain management doctor's monitoring system and behave like a perfect patient. There are even websites selling fake urine powder for people to put in warm water to give to doctors, pretending these are their own samples!

What if the urine samples need to be collected and monitored on the spot? This, by the way, would mean that somebody would have to watch this patient pee in the cup. No worries. The internet sells penises in all colors and shapes which are connected to a reservoir of reconstituted fake urine. The male patient could place the fake penis between his legs and squeeze the warm yellow liquid into the cup in front of the monitor. The urine would smell like the real thing. It would be warm as if it were produced from a human body because the reservoir would be kept right next to the warm skin.

If there are so many loopholes and ways for patients to cheat the system, what is the point of doing the monitoring? This is not a perfect system. We do our best to encourage patients to do the right thing and follow all appropriate guidelines to reduce risk of medication misuse or overdose. When I hand over an opioid prescription to a patient, the piece of paper carries much more weight than it seems. It carries the trust in the patient to follow instructions and use the medication responsibly. It also carries a doctor's legal and ethical liability for providing this potentially lethal substance.

Even though I would like to understand and monitor all my patients' opioid use, it is an unattainable goal.

For example, if I gave out a prescription of oxycodone, 5mg one tablet every eight hours, for fourteen days, the patient would take home forty-two pills. I could never be certain my direction is how the patient would use the pills. He could take all forty-two pills at the same time and die from an over dosage, from my prescription. The only way to verify that he follows my prescription directions is to accompany this patient home and personally watch him swallow a pill every eight hours. This would be unfeasible. As physicians, we monitor patients' behavior as best we can. On the other hand, our patients are capable adults who make their own choices. How much responsibility do we, should we, or can we take, for our patients?

ONE OF MY pain management colleagues had a patient who had been taking morphine 15mg, which was the lowest dosage morphine pills available on the market. She would take one pill, twice a day for her chronic pain and had been receiving a monthly supply of sixty pills. For years, she remained stable without behavioral problems.

One morning, she was found dead in her bed of an apparent suicide. The patient's husband called my colleague and blamed his wife's death on him:

"She died only because she took the whole bottle of morphine pills. You gave her the pills!"

"You killed my wife! Wait for my lawyer to call. I'll see you in court."

Fortunately, my colleague was never sued, but at times like this, we all feel disheartened, sad, and deeply stressed. We well understood the husband's grief and anger. However, in reality, how can we monitor and guarantee a patient to follow our instructions without deviation? How can doctors possibly be expected to pick up signs of depression and suicide when the closest people in a patient's life cannot even succeed in doing so?

Risk of physical harm and of legal trouble sometimes take the pleasure out of my daily role of being a physician, a job that I love. I try to look at the bright side and ignore the negatives. Yet there are times that it haunts me.

It is, after all, a risky business.

"However you disguise it, this thing does not change: The perpetual struggle of Good and Evil." — T.S. Eliot

I STOP
A Means to Prevent Controlled Substances From Being Over-Prescribed

THE STATE OF New York unveiled the "Internet System for Tracking Over-Prescribing," or I STOP in 2012. The New York State Legislature unanimously passed it and was signed into law in August of 2012. New York became the first state in the nation to mandate that physicians consult an Internet database containing a patient's prescription history before prescribing a schedule II, III, or IV controlled substance.

These enhancements of the state's Prescription Monitoring Program (PMP) are invaluable in providing doctors with a patient's accurate and up-to-date controlled substance history. It helps to eliminate the problem of stolen and forged prescriptions being used to obtain controlled substances from pharmacies. It cracks down on illegal "doctor shopping"—the practice of visiting several different doctors and pharmacies for controlled prescription drugs.

I was very excited about the I STOP program. Finally, I could STOP making those phone calls to pharmacies to verify patient prescriptions. I could also eliminate a large amount of correspondence with other doctors because the entire history of patient's opioid and controlled substance use would already be available in the system.

This program can be used by doctors and pharmacists to identify patterns of abuse; and to accurately prescribe medication and other controlled substances to patients who truly need them. At the same time, it arms medical professionals with the necessary data to detect potentially dangerous drug interactions, such as the dual use of opioids and benzodiazepines (Valium, Xanax, and such) which can put patients at higher risk of respiratory depression. With I STOP, a new world appeared for me and my colleagues. Or, I should say, we had the key to open a world that we could not see before. A few of my patients were evidently getting opioids from multiple providers, as shown in the I STOP system. By then, I was no longer surprised by anything I saw, but I was still somewhat amazed by some of the results shown.

One patient had been with me for many years without any known problems. She would bring every office staff member a holiday present every year. She would share her stories of her children with us. We all felt like she was one of us, like family, until it turned out that she was doctor shopping.

The saddest story of all was that the seemingly most loving, caring grandma we treated was caught selling her multiple prescription opioids for grocery money, as she claimed.

All of them appeared to have above board behavior before I STOP revealed the truth. I had to discharge them and send them for detox and rehabilitation.

I STOP, in addition, allowed me to have a glimpse of how other physicians prescribed opioids.

Danny, a young man in his twenties, showed up in my office, complaining of chronic foot pain due to a sports injury which did not heal properly after surgery. I checked his I STOP, which indicated that he received twelve hundred pills of oxycodone 20mg in the past month! That would be forty pills of 20mg oxycodone each day. This amount is almost twenty to thirty times of what I usually would prescribe to my patients.

"This must be a mistake," I thought. "It is probably a hundred and twenty pills which would still be an extraordinary amount. The last zero had to be a mistake."

Since the information in I STOP was entered by the pharmacists when the medications were dispensed, I thought it might have been a clerical error, made by the pharmacy staff. I called the druggist to verify the information.

"It was one thousand and two hundred pills that the patient got," the pharmacist who took my call said. "I know, it was such a ridiculous amount. I, myself, called the prescribing physician to confirm that was really what he wanted to prescribe."

My jaw dropped and hit the floor. I was in astonishment long after I hung up the phone. What kind of doctor would give the patient such an enormous number of opioids? I looked up the prescribing physician and learned that he was a psychiatrist who started the patient on a low dose of oxycodone about eight months before. In the past six months, he managed to increase the total narcotic prescription by two hundred-fold. I could not produce any rationale to medically explain this need.

"Yes, doctor, I know I have a big problem," Danny told me as soon as I walked into the consultation room.

"I am taking about twelve pills of oxycodone every day. That is why I am here. I need help."

Danny appeared straightforward. He started talking before I did. I was unequivocal with him. I explained that what he needed was a detox center, not a doctor who would continue to provide opioids for him. I sent him away with information about local drug detox centers and ones that were farther afield.

After he left, I caught myself thinking, Wait a minute. Didn't he say he took twelve pills a day? He never said he took forty pills a day. So, he would have only used 360 pills for the month. What did he do with the leftover of 840 pills? Each pill was 20mg. He would have a total of 16,800mg of extra oxycodone per month. The market price for oxycodone was one dollar per milligram. That would mean he could pocket $16,800 if he had sold them. If he had sold everything on the street, his income last month would have been $24,000, which would have been tax free!

Nice little entrepreneurship there, Danny.

> "Nothing ever turns out the way we expect, good or bad."
> — Matthew May

Phoebe and the Red Flag

WHEN PHOEBE CAME in for her monthly medication refill of methadone, her I-STOP printout indicated that she had picked up a prescription of sixty pills of oxycodone from another doctor. Obtaining pain medications from any other physician would be a breach to her narcotics contract and it was caught by the I STOP process. I was not happy to find this out, especially since I trusted Phoebe, who should have known better after coming to my office for so many years.

When I showed the I STOP printout to Phoebe, she sadly said, "I had another knee surgery, Dr. Shue. Believe me, I told the surgeon that I did not want any pain medication because I have my own pain management doctor. The office called them in anyway even without telling me about it. I have been your patient for so many years. I know the rules. I never asked for them, I swear. The orthopedist just called them in automatically after patients' surgeries."

I felt sad and sorry for Phoebe. I was not convinced by what she told me. I knew her orthopedist had been treating her since the time she was a drug abuser. I was confident that no physician would ever call in any controlled substance without a patient's request, especially when the physician had the knowledge of her chronic pain and history of substance abuse.

I had to call the orthopedist's office to verify Phoebe's dishonesty.

"Yes, we called in the oxycodone as a routine practice after her surgery."

The office staff looked through Phoebe's chart and confirmed on the phone.

"Did you have any record that the patient had requested the prescription?" I asked.

"No, the patient did not request it."

What could I say? I was appalled and upset at how generous some of the physicians were, giving out opioids. Pain management physicians use opioids frequently. We understand the use of controlled substance can easily become out of control. All health care providers need to be on the same page.

Interventional pain management physicians, like myself, probably use opioids most sparingly. We prefer to use interventional procedures and injections to improve patients' pain.

Narcotics management is only a small part of our practices. The truth of the matter is that we, as specialists, can allay the patient's pain and fear with many other treatments. Yet, many people come to us specifically for opioid treatment. Some doctors simply tell their patients, "I don't feel comfortable giving you opioids anymore. See a pain management doctor to take over your prescriptions."

When the requirement of ISTOP started, some doctors decided that it was not worthwhile to mess around with the new laws and regulations. They decided to leave narcotic prescribing out of their practices. However, when patients only expected to have their previous prescription continued, it was often difficult to convince them to consider the many other treatment options to quell their pain.

Phoebe had already left when I called her orthopedist's office. I pulled my office manager aside to make sure we red-flagged Phoebe's chart and we would obtain a urine toxicology screen for the next few visits.

Even though the oxycodone prescription was called in without Phoebe's request, she did not have to pick it up. She chose to purchase it from the pharmacy and took it home. No patient would be forced to pick up a prescription. She could have argued that she did not pay attention to what she had picked up along with all her other medications. She still should not have consumed any oxycodone if she were to follow my directions. I wanted to see if Phoebe were using oxycodone which would show up in her urine toxicology study.

THE FOLLOWING MONTH, Phoebe's urine toxicology results came back. She was negative for oxycodone use, but her urine was positive for cocaine! My heart sank when I saw the results. Really? All these years of being sober? Or was she really sober as she claimed? Was she just that good cheating the system, and me?

Phoebe would not tell me when she started using street drugs again. I was furious at Phoebe for letting herself down yet again after all her struggles and suffering. It finally came down to the necessary confrontation. I gave her information of drug rehabilitation programs, wished her luck, and discharged her from my practice.

I have a zero-tolerance policy. Every patient has to respect and follow the narcotics contract. No exceptions.

"A straight foot has no fear of a crooked shoe." — Chinese proverb

Melissa, the Whistleblower

One afternoon, Melissa came for her medication refill. Melissa, a thirty-something mother, was passed onto me by another physician. She was taking chronic high dosage of opioids for her severe neck, low back spine and nerve pain, despite multiple spine surgeries. Surgeons all deemed her not suitable for further surgical intervention. I had been giving her steroid injections to minimize her discomfort, while tapering down her opioid use.

Melissa stood up abruptly as I entered the consultation room. She reached out to grab my hand and pulled me closer.

"Dr. Shue, I recognized that woman outside in the waiting room. I know where she lives. That entire building is full of terrible people. I know it because my brother used to live there. I went to that building often before my brother died, and I saw that woman there. She sells her morphine pills. She asked me to sell her my morphine pills too.

"Do you know who I am talking about? I don't know this woman's name. She has a disabled daughter. Everyone in that building knows her. Believe me, I am a highly educated person and I don't lie. I used to work as a paralegal in a high-caliber law firm before my disability curtailed my opportunity to work.

"That woman is dangerous. You need to get rid of her. Don't tell anyone that I told you this. It will get me in a lot of trouble. Those are bad, bad people. They are going to hurt me if they find out what I just told you. They might hurt you too."

I knew right away that Melissa was referring to Julie. Julie was a middle-aged single mom of a seven-year-old-daughter with cerebral palsy. Julie was on social security disability because of severe psoriatic arthritis and lupus. She lived in a government-subsidized housing building and had been my patient for three years. She appeared to be one of those no trouble, stable, on minimal narcotic dosage type of patients.

Frequently, Julie would bring her daughter with her in a wheelchair because she did not have available childcare. Julie lamented one Halloween that her daughter had no trick or treat candies because there was nowhere they could go, living in an apartment building in a bad neighborhood. Ever since then, I set aside a drawer of candy in my office. Every time Julie's daughter came in, she could trick or treat with us.

After I heard what Melissa told me, I felt slightly helpless. I was numbed after finding out yet another long term "good" patient, turned out to be an excellent con-artist. I no longer understood whether my patients were too good at grifting, if they just that desperate, or if I was just too foolish to know better.

When I saw Julie in the office later that day, I suggested that we change her generic morphine to a new formulation of brand name morphine with an abuse deterrent technology. The new morphine pills are formulated with inactive ingredients that make the tablet more difficult to adulterate for misuse and abuse, even if the tablets were subjected to physical manipulation and/or chemical extraction.

Compared to traditional morphine tablets, these new pills, as least claimed by the pharmaceutical company, increased resistance to cutting and crushing. When put in any liquid, the medication would form a viscous material that would not be passed through a needle. If Julie was, indeed, selling her morphine pills, the new pills would have much less street value. Then she would likely come back to me and request to be put on her previous pills.

Julie did not object to the change of her morphine, even when I explained to her the reason for the change was to decrease the street value of my patients' prescription medications. In fact, she was happy about the pills over the next few months. Her I STOP and urine toxicology results were all appropriate.

When Melissa blew the whistle on Julie, it reminded me about how Phoebe ratted out Tim and Jack. It took me a long time to catch Phoebe using an illicit substance. This made me wonder if Phoebe had squealed on the two brothers to be righteous, or, had she been proactive to get rid of Tim and Jack to prevent them from disclosing her own inappropriate behavior?

In Melissa's case, did Melissa really see Julie selling drugs? Or, was Melissa afraid that Julie would say something about her own problems?

For months since I started keeping an eye on both, Melissa and Phoebe had clean records and lab results. Feedback from their primary care physicians did not show any red flags either. Who was the real problematic patient? One or both? Whom, if any, should I usher out of my practice?

"A straight foot has no fear of a crooked shoe." The Chinese proverb means that those conduct themselves with honesty and integrity need not fear others' gossip and accusation. Time will tell. I will be patient.

It is exhausting to play private eye, while being a full-time physician. I have nowhere to turn to find answers. Not even I STOP can do its magic one hundred percent of the time.

When I STOP and all paper trails fail to show any behavior problems, family members and friends sometimes become the last lifeline we have.

One day, a staff member put her hand over the phone speaker and said, "Dr. Shue, your patient Gail's father requested to speak to you. It's urgent."

She connected me with Gail's father, John. His daughter had a large lumbar herniated disc a year before, and she had surgery to correct the problem. Her pain initially improved but became severe again in recent months. She planned to have another spine surgery for the pain, but she was waiting to sort out a health care insurance issue first.

Gail continued to work with me and had lumbar epidural injections a few times, but they did not help. Reluctantly, I gave her two pills of 5mg oxycodone each day, a total of sixty pills for the month while waiting for her to have the second surgery.

Then the call from Gail's father came.

"Thanks for taking my call, Doctor. I know you are under a patient confidentiality agreement and cannot talk to me about my daughter. I just need you to listen to me. You don't need to say a word to break the agreement."

He paused and said, "Gail has been abusing oxycodone. She has taken all sixty pills you gave her in just a few days. Then she went to buy more on the street to get high. She would not listen to us when we told her we knew all about her problem.

"Her husband said he will be taking the kids and he will leave her if she doesn't do something about it—now. This has been going on for the past two months, ever since her low back pain got worse. We need your help. Please talk to her when she comes to your office next time. Maybe you can convince her that she needs to go to a rehab center to detox. We tried, but she would not listen to us. We are so afraid that we would find her dead one day."

John started crying. It was heart breaking to hear an elderly father fall apart on the phone over his adult child.

It turned out that Gail agreed to go to the detox program soon after the phone call, without my intervention. Gail was lucky. She had concerned family members who cared about her and took initiatives to get her the help she needed.

I wish all my patients had friends and family members who could be my eyes and ears outside of my office to watch the patients for me. If they notice patients abusing drugs, or if they misuse their medications, they could report to me. Then I would know exactly to whom I should prescribe opioids, how much to prescribe, and whom I should say no to, with absolute confidence. Just think of the decisions I had to make concerning Tim, Jack, Phoebe, Melissa, and Julie? It's a whirlwind of conscience-raising decisions and sometimes it lingers in my mind long after I have left the office.

"A comfort zone is a beautiful place. But nothing ever grows there."
— John Assaraf

Training, Trying

DURING MY TRAINING in the late 1990s and 2000s, this is what I was taught:

If a doctor prescribed a patient an opioid for relief from pain for surgery or chronic disease, it was unlikely one would need to worry unless the patient had existing addiction issues. It's extremely rare for people who do not already have substance abuse problems to become addicted to pain medication.

As physicians, we always feel obligated to do something—anything—to reduce patients' suffering. We do not want to overlook a patient's report of pain. The letter published in the New England Journal of Medicine on January 10, 1980, provided physicians a new comfort level as they prescribed opioids to patients. We were taught from then on, that the stigma on narcotics was unfounded and patients should not suffer when there were medications readily available to improve their quality of life.

The Joint Commission first established standards for pain assessment and treatment in 2001, in response to the national outcry about the widespread problem of undertreatment of painful issues.

The CMS (Centers for Medicare and Medicaid Services) used the HCAHPS (Hospital Consumer Assessment of Healthcare Providers and Systems) survey to help determine health care facility performances. This survey was the first national, standardized, publicly reported perspective of hospital care. Pain-related questions from HCAHPS, were used to determine hospital reimbursement rates.

The survey included three specific questions. It asked:

1. Whether patients needed medication for pain
2. If their pain were well controlled during their stay
3. If the hospital staff did "everything they could" to help with their pain[1]

Linking hospital performance and reimbursements to patient satisfaction with pain treatment, led to encouragement for the extensive treatment of pain. Doctors and hospitals were penalized if they didn't treat patient's pain well enough and they let patients suffer.

---

1   https://www.cms.gov/Medicare/Quality-Initiatives-Patient-Assessment-Instruments/HospitalQualityInits/HospitalHCAHPS

During my training as a resident and fellow physician, the majority of my professors were comfortable using high dose opioids for chronically ill patients. A daily dosage of 200 to 300mg OxyContin or more, was common. It was also widely believed that if a patient developed tolerance toward a pain medication, dosages needed to be raised by about fifty percent to be effective.

For example, if a patient were using morphine, 200mg daily, but pain was not controlled, the dosage would be increased to 300mg daily. Any less of an increase would only result in the body building up tolerance. It would be ineffective to control pain.

We recognized that the human body would get used to pain medication. Over time, the drugs would become ineffective. Then we would implement narcotic rotation. We would switch the patient to another kind of opioid in order for the body to use a new chemical that would likely to be more effective.

Patients, were nonetheless, maintained on chronic narcotics. High dosages of narcotic use, although not preferred, were acceptable as a reasonable treatment choice.

As much as modern medicine had evolved, there were limitations. I saw it every day in my practice. No single treatment modality could manage everyone's medical conditions.

I clearly realized that some patients were unable to manage their pain without pharmacological treatments, despite interventional pain management injections. My own reaction was to assuage the pain in any way I could, and sometimes opioids held the key.

"The development of addiction is rare in medical patients with no history of addiction."

I read and reread these well-remembered words. If the big names at the New England Journal of Medicine didn't worry, and if my professors were comfortable using narcotics in high dosages, I decided not to be scared of them either. If my patients who were on high dosages of narcotics, truly needed the medication, then they needed doctors like me to help them reduce their suffering to live a functional life.

I diligently used all the tools I had to monitor my patients. Narcotic contracts, random urine toxicology testing, pill counting, communication between pharmacies and other physicians were implemented with all my narcotic patients. I was proud to have a strict and clean pain management practice.

Unfortunately, what I learned and saw in the Ivory Tower of training definitely did not prepare me well enough for the real world. My good intentions of providing patients with quality care did not exempt me from getting tangled up with problematic results. Before long, patients like Tim, Jack, Phoebe, and Danny, just to name a few, managed to provide me with eye opening experiences. They showed me how deep, dark, complicated, and hurtful overuse and misuse of narcotics could become.

Even though my narcotic-using patients consist of a small percentage of my practice, I increasingly found that the majority of my daily work-related stress stemmed from managing them. Some of my colleagues did not see this as being a worthwhile endeavor, either financially, logistically, or legally. They quickly changed their offices to interventional pain management only, meaning that they only offered procedures, not opioids management.

Should I also change my practice to only use procedures, non-opioid medications, but not narcotics? Or should I still offer patients the full spectrum of pain management options? If so, how could I do it in a safe way?

While I was unsure about my answer as to the direction of my own practice, evidently, other physicians were also seeing the problems of opioid use and weighing the same decisions.

David Juurlick, a Toronto physician who reported in 2017, said that opioids are problematic for all users.

He said, "Opioids really do afford relief—initially—but that relief tends to diminish over time.[2] That's, in part, why people increase their dosage. They are chasing pain relief from a drug that fails in the long run.

"I see many people who are convinced they are legitimate patients. They are on massive doses of opioids, and they are telling me that they need this medication, which is clearly doing them harm, over time. The primary benefit of therapy at this point becomes not going into withdrawal."

In 2016 alone, over 50,000 Americans died from opioid overdoses, while another 20.5 million were heavily addicted to the drugs.

Over the course of modern American history, more people have died from opioid drug overuse than from wars, and motor vehicle accidents. These statistics are based on data from the Centers for Disease Control and reported in Prevention magazine in 2017.

Between April of 2020 to April 2021, according to data released from the CDC, over 100,000 Americans died of drug overdoses. Now, it is clearly evident that this opioid epidemic has gotten out of control.

"The opioid epidemic is this generation's AIDS crisis," Andrew Sullivan reported in New York Magazine.[3]

How did this happen? People suddenly woke up from this nightmare and started asking questions and pointing fingers.

Some said it was the pharmaceutical industry's financial greed that drove narcotics to be promoted in a way to mislead physicians to prescribe them,

2   https://www.cfr.org/backgrounder/us-opioid-epidemic
3   https://nymag.com/intelligencer/2017/03/the-opioid-epidemic-is-this-generations-aids-crisis.html

thinking they were safer than they really were. Some said it was physicians' own thirst for cash, resulting in unethical narcotic pill mills, distributing opioids to the masses.

In addition, regulatory guidelines played a role too. Some doctors and experts, think that the Joint Commission's Management Standards helped grow the idea of pain as a "fifth vital sign." [4]It required healthcare providers to ask every patient about their pain and encouraged the use of medication.

The Joint Commission's current standards actually require that organizations establish policies regarding pain assessment and treatment and conduct educational efforts to ensure compliance. The standards do not require the use of drugs to manage a patient's pain and when a drug is appropriate, the standards do not specify which drugs should be prescribed.

Nobody wants to take the blame for the national opioid crisis. No single force could have resulted in this massive problem. It had to be multifactorial to form this perfect storm. However, the problem still needs to be urgently addressed.

In 2016, the Centers for Disease Control in Atlanta, Georgia came out with recommendations entitled "Determining When to Initiate or Continue Opioids for Chronic Pain."

The CDC said when opioids are started, doctors should prescribe the lowest effective dosage, and should use caution when using opioids at any dosage. Doctors should carefully reassess each patient's benefits and risks when considering increasing dosage to more than fifty morphine milligram equivalents (MME) per day. They should avoid increasing dosage to more than ninety MME per day. Higher doses of opioids are associated with higher risk of overdose and death. Even relatively low doses (twenty-to-fifty morphine milligram equivalents (MME) per day) increased risk. Previous guidelines focused safety precautions on "high risk patients." The new guidelines remind doctors that opioids pose risk to all patients, and currently available tools cannot effectively tell doctors what kind of patients are safe from risks and problems related to opioid use[5].

The CDC noted that the benefits of high-dose opioids for chronic pain are not established, but that risks for serious harm, related to opioid therapy, increases at higher opioid dosage. Specifically, the Guideline notes that most experts generally agreed that increasing dosages to fifty or more MME per day increases overdose risk without necessarily adding benefits for pain control or function.

Because each opioid has a different potency, Milligram Morphine Equivalent (MME) is a value assigned to different opioids to represent their

4	https://www.medpagetoday.com/publichealthpolicy/publichealth/57336#
5	https://www.cdc.gov/mmwr/volumes/65/

relative potencies. MME is determined by using an equivalency factor to calculate a dose of an opioid that is equivalent to morphine. For instance, 65mg oxycodone, 25mg hydromorphone, and 37mcg/hr of fentanyl patch all have about the same morphine equivalent which equals 100mg. In other words, all of the above medications should work similarly on a patient in terms of pain relief and side effects. This way, doctors, pharmacies, and patients all have a reference point of how much opioid a patient is on no matter which specific medication he or she is taking.

Patients often ask me which opioid is stronger. The short answer is that any single one opioid can be "stronger" if it is taken in a higher MME dosage. If a patient takes 100mg of morphine a day, it is as strong as taking 65mg of oxycodone.

After the CDC guidelines came out, the Center of Medicare and Medicaid services and insurance companies followed and released their recommendations for opioid prescription guidelines. Some insurance companies placed a restriction to the number of pills or amount of total Milligram Morphine Equivalent a patient can obtain each month. If a patient needs a higher amount, the treating physician has to fill out extra paperwork to explain why the patient requires more, and if all measurements are used to ensure safety of the medication use.

I usually see these rules and regulations as interference with our autonomy and ability to providing the best care for patients. The paperwork alone, adds stress and overhead to a physician's office and reduces patient care time. However, this time, I welcomed the new regulations.

There are many different opinions and reactions toward the CDC guidelines regarding opioid use. In general, they can be categorized into two sides. On one side, people believe that when opioids are taken long term at high dosages, patients' body get so tolerant, the medications no longer work. Worse, it can result in Opioid-induced hyperalgesia. This means, the more pain medication one is taking, the more sensitive the person is going to be to painful stimuli and therefore would feel more pain. Most likely, more medications will be required to calm down the worsened pain. The only way to stop this vicious cycle is to wean off the opioids all together. Once the receptors in the body are normalized with time, low dose pain medication would work again.

On the other hand, some people recognize the tolerance and potential risks associated with chronic high dosage opioid use. However, they argue, patients would not be able to function or lead a meaningful or productive life if pain relief is taken away. Taking opioids would be the less of the evil. Therefore, it is reasonable to continue high dose opioid therapy.

I believe the value of chronic opioid treatment, but I am not convinced that high dosage opioid use is beneficial to patient's pain management long term. Over the years, I tried to encourage my patients to decrease their opioid dosage, but my efforts had been met with much resistance and failure. The CDC guidelines and the new rules developed by insurance companies can help me motivate my patients to taper down their narcotic use.

I decided to start with patients who were on opioid dosages more than 90mg morphine equivalent (MME) per day, because the CDC guidelines clearly state that any dosage at or above this should be avoided. I set aside extra time to counsel these patients regarding the reasons and benefits for the narcotic dosage change. I promised them that their medication would be tapered down gradually each month in the span of three to six months.

This gentle change would prevent withdrawal syndrome to any degree. It would also decrease patient anxiety and increase success rate. Once the body has a new baseline of opioid intake, it would adjust to it.

When I made the decision to undergo this opioid weaning endeavor, I fully expected my patients to fight with me and call me ugly names. I warned my office staff regarding the possible yelling and screaming coming from within the office. On occasions, I even had a staff member standing outside of my consultation room as my bodyguard, anticipating the conversation with the patient turned sour and violent.

I got just what I expected. I had patients shouting, "I am going to die from pain. It is all because you stupid doctors don't want to do the right thing to give me what I need! If you don't give this to me, I'm going to go on the street to get drugs, and it's all your fault. I wish you would become so sick with horrible pain, so you'd know exactly how it feels to be me."

What I heard the most was, "Aren't you supposed to be a pain management doctor? What good are you if you don't give me my pills?"

Patients would give me nasty stares, curse, whip open the consultation room door and stomp out of my office, slamming the front door behind them. Some vowed never to return. Some never did.

Luckily, we never had to use our bodyguard.

I understood why "not enough" had been done by physicians to oppose the opioid epidemic. From a physicians' standpoint, it would be so much easier to hand patients prescriptions for the supply of another month of pain medications. Patients would be happy, easy going, and life would go on. The office visit would be quick and pleasant. It would be much more exhausting and time consuming to try to lower the amount or refuse medication and explain to patients why I do so.

Still, I routinely hear:

"Why fix it when it is not broken?"

"My life has been so stable during the past ten years while I take my medicine. What are you trying to do here?

"How am I going to function at work, play with my children or even be a normal human being?"

"I don't care what studies or statistics say. I am an individual patient, and my needs may not be the same as the scientific paper results."

"I am not abusing any medication. I don't want to be dependent on them, but I need them."

These were not easy statements or questions to handle, especially for patients who have had multiple spine or joint surgeries, who tried everything else for their pain control. What evidence did I have to assure them that their lives would not be affected using less opioids? They were not taking them for recreational use. They were, indeed, trying to live a normal life—as normal as possible.

Yes, every single patient needed to be evaluated as an individual. Which individual needed more? How much more? How would I determine these issues?

As I struggled to learn from the process itself and figure out how to help my patients wean down their opioid use, I discovered that a reasonable number of my patients were surprisingly agreeable to the plan to reduce what they were currently taking.

I initially focused on weaning my patients to a lower daily dosage. For some of them, it went so smoothly, that they actually asked to keep on going to reduce the amount.

Bob, who was a quiet and reserved man in his sixties started to come see me. His wife would accompany him on every visit. When I first saw him in the consultation room, he struck me as somewhat peculiar, but I could not put my finger on it. His eyes were dim, and his face was flat, blatantly apathetic.

Paula did all the talking. Bob just stared straight into space, as if the conversation between his wife and I had nothing to do with him.

"Bob has been suffering from constant abdominal pain for many years, His primary care physician has done all kinds of tests but could not figure out why he suffers so much. They sent him to pain management doctors all over the area. For the past five years, he was put on narcotic medications with different names that I can't even remember. The doses kept going up and up, but his pain is still so bad. He can't even sleep. Every time he eats or goes to the bathroom, the pain is worse because he has terrible constipation. We are at our wits end. A friend of ours told us about you, so here we are, trying our luck once again."

Paula pulled out a stack of papers, detailing the MRIs, CT scans, ultrasounds, endoscopies, colonoscopies, and lab results performed throughout the years, all of which were normal. The diagnosis written on Bob's chart was "idiopathic abdominal pain," which essentially meant that his doctors did not know why he had stomach pain.

The good news was that nothing life-threatening or serious was going on in Bob's abdomen. Nonetheless, this was not good enough for Bob, because he still experienced pain every day. The lack of identifiable pathology unfortunately did not translate into a lack of discomfort.

In the era of modern medicine, lacking a real diagnosis that can explain one's symptoms can be very frustrating, disturbing, and outright unacceptable for patients. Healthcare providers have to constantly remind patients and ourselves that no matter how many breakthroughs have been achieved over the years, the secrets and mysteries of the human body are so enormous. Some are still beyond human comprehension. Every new discovery leads to new questions, and this will be an endless endeavor, which makes medicine an exciting and intriguing profession.

Bob and Paula seemed to have made peace with the lack of a "real" diagnosis. They just wanted him to suffer less. Bob was originally started on a low dosage of opioids for his pain. Over a span of five years, he tried many different types of opioids, and his oxycodone dosage was increased to 80mg, three times a day by the time he came to see me.

Bob was a tough patient to treat. The lack of pathology and the generalized nature of his abdominal pain meant that the nerve blocks and injections I frequently use were inappropriate for him. The main focus of his treatment would have to include behavioral therapy and medication adjustment.

I discussed the importance of having a psychologist or a psychiatrist involved to treat possible depression, which I suspected, given Bob's flat facial affect. I encouraged Bob to pay attention to exercise and healthful dietary choices.

Lastly, I explained, "High dosage of opioids are actually not indicated for non-cancer pain, which is fortunate in my case. We all know that taking opioids can make people feel better, especially at the beginning. However, with time, as the brain gets used to the medication, the body demands more and more. A high dosage of opioids can sometimes lead to side effects which can be more problematic than the problem we are treating or the potential benefits of the drug.

"As you know, Paula, Bob has severe constipation, which is in all likelihood, making his abdominal distress even worse. The high dosage of oxycodone probably is what gave him the terrible bowel problem. I know it sounds counterintuitive, but I would like Bob to start cutting back on his oxycodone."

Paula looked at me, then she looked at Bob, who blinked his eyes but did not move his facial muscles or say anything to express his thoughts.

"It's funny you said that." Paula raised her eyebrows. "It all kind of makes sense to me. Bob didn't look like this before. I often wonder myself if he is taking too much oxycodone, which is putting him in this mental fog all day. I did not want to take the medication away from him, fearing that he would be in worse pain, but now that you suggested it, I can't agree with you more. But would he go into any withdrawal or more problems if you take away the pain pills?"

I did not expect that Paula was ready to take on the plan with such enthusiasm. Then it dawned on me why Bob looked different. How could I have overlooked this side effect of oxycodone? He did look like he was in a "mental fog," as described by his wife.

I assured Paula and Bob that I would taper him down very slowly to avoid withdrawal problems, although he might still feel some mild discomfort every time his opioid dosage was reduced. We agreed that Bob would come to see me monthly for follow-up and further weaning of his medication.

With Paula's determination and Bob's motivation, the weaning process went very smoothly. When Bob's medication was reduced to two-thirds of his original dosage, Paula told me excitedly, "Bob is doing much better and seems to be almost like himself again. He seems to be more awake during the day, with more energy. He even smiles more and talks more now. Right? Bob?"

Paula elbowed Bob, who blinked and chuckled slightly with a shy expression. With further weaning of his oxycodone, Bob's pain remained an issue, but he was stable. His constipation dramatically improved. He started on a low-dose antidepressant recommended by his new psychiatrist. He also began to attend chronic pain support group meetings every week.

Paula was happy that her husband was back to himself, no longer in the constant mental fog. Bob's idiopathic abdominal pain was still there, bothering him every day. However, he had learned to cope with it. Getting off his high dose of oxycodone did not exactly help his pain, but it did not make it worse. Most importantly, it took away the side effects that were associated with chronic high dose opioid therapy. Overall, it made a tremendous improvement in his quality of life.

Almost every day, I used success stories, such as Bob's, to encourage other people to wean down their opioid use as much as possible. It was not always as smooth or as exciting a process each time. Most of my patients advanced and then they regressed, back and forth—back and forth. I had to negotiate with them, set new goals and make new plans as situations evolved.

It was frustrating and demoralizing at times. Patients sometimes had bursts of anger, questioning again and again why I would stir up trouble in their lives. I would sink into doubt and question if all the effort was worthwhile.

With time, more and more patients stopped and said, "Dr. Shue. Thank you so much for your help to push me through this process. It's sometimes harder than I believe it could ever be, but it's all worth it."

"Don't thank me, you are the one who did it, not me," I reply.

"But Dr. Shue, you were the first doctor who took the time to talk to me and encourage me, instead of just giving me yet another prescription refill and send me out of the door," one patient said to me.

My patients' kind words are the ultimate recognition for my continual effort and struggle to reduce the use of high-dose opioids in my patient population Their encouragement heaves me out of my comfort zone and motivates me to plow on toward the right direction, even if that isn't the easiest path.

"Crossing the river by touching the stones." — Ancient Chinese Folk Saying

Liz: A Case of Severe Overuse . . . or Not?

WHEN LIZ CAME to my office the first time, I was swamped. She had to wait more than half an hour. When it was her turn to be seen, I had to run to the bathroom first. It is hard for people to imagine why doctors do not even have time to go the restroom. I did not want to get myself in this embarrassing situation either. Yet, I had been running into consult room after consult room with no breaks all day, not wanting my patients to wait for me. I just could not stand it anymore. Liz had to wait.

As I walked out of the rest room, Liz was walking out of her consult room.

"Hi, Liz, I am Dr. Shue. I'm so sorry you had to wait so long. Why don't we go back to the room so we can see what I can do for you?"

"No, I have to go now. I don't have time. I've waited for too long. Your staff told me that you went to the restroom, and I needed to wait, but I can't wait for a doctor who rather go to the rest room than see me first."

Liz sized me up and was obviously unhappy. Truthfully, I would also be annoyed if I had to wait this long. It wasn't her fault that it hadn't occurred to her that doctors still needed to take care of their basic needs, even in the midst of a busy workday. In fact, I have heard similar complaints, even from my own friends.

"I am here for my terrible low back pain and sciatica. But now I will have to figure out what to do myself."

Liz stopped in the hallway, turned to me, and proceeded to keep talking about her pain for the next five minutes.

"If you don't mind, I can quickly review your MRI results, do a physical exam, and then tell you what can be done to make you feel better."

Liz spent yet another ten minutes telling me more about her ailment, still in the hallway. Then she declared, ignoring my repeat invitation for a formal evaluation in the consultation room, while walking toward the exit, "The stars just did not line up today. I knew something wasn't right for me. I may or may not come back, depending on what my heart tells me to do."

One month later, Liz's heart must have told her to return to my office. Or maybe it was that the stars aligned. Or her pain eventually gained a bigger voice than her heart or the stars. This time around I promptly reviewed her chart and did not dare to delay.

Due to a deteriorating lumbar disc disease and life-long scoliosis, Liz, at age fifty-five, was taking a large dose of morphine. Liz's back issues had been managed by her primary physician. When a large amount of opioids could not reduce her pain, her doctor sent her to me for further diagnosis and treatment.

I discussed treatment options with Liz. She suffered with severe spine pathology and likely would need surgery. I referred her to be evaluated by a spine surgeon, who explained to her that corrective spine surgery would definitely be needed. With that information, she decided to undergo the required procedure within the year.

"Dr. Shue, my surgery has been scheduled. Before I have my surgery, I need you to help me keep my pain under control. My pain pills aren't working anymore." Liz said to me during her follow up appointment.

"Liz, you need to start taking less opioid medications," I told her. "You have been taking too much opioid drugs for far too long. Your body is used to them and that is why they do not work well anymore. If you keep taking this amount of opioids, it would be difficult to have your pain under control after surgery when you experience more pain from the surgical trauma and healing."

Liz was taking a total of 800mg morphine equivalent per day. She definitely had narcotic tolerance. I explained to Liz the new CDC guideline regarding chronic opioid use. My goal was to cut her back as close to 90mg morphine equivalent as possible, as the CDC guideline suggested.

The FDA defines a patient like Liz, as opioid tolerant if he or she has been receiving oral morphine 60mg each day for at least one week, or the equivalent dose of any other opioids.

Opioid tolerance implies that a patient would feel less effects of the drugs—both relief and side effects—and it may develop in people with long-term use of the medications. Patients who are prescribed opioids for management of chronic pain, or who have an opioid addiction may all become opioid tolerant.

When there is a new injury to the body, such as traumatic surgical incisions, the patient develops acute pain. It can be very challenging to manage acute pain in patients with opioid tolerance, because the medications that usually help after surgery, become ineffective in these patients. Therefore, if the amount of opioid consumption can be reduced before surgery, it would be helpful for patient's overall pain management, especially after surgery.

Liz was far from thrilled with the idea of taking less medication.

"How can I function with a reduction of my pills? I can barely do anything, as is, while taking all my pills. Most of the day, I could use even more pills."

With my perseverance, she reluctantly gave in.

"I am a very spiritual person. I pray every day. In fact, I pray a lot. I had a sense that you are a very spiritual person too. God tells me that you will take good care of me. I am going to try to follow your plan."

Liz did fine slowly reducing her daily morphine from 800mg to 400mg. Things took an one hundred eighty degree turn when I tried to decrease her medication from a daily dosage of 400mg to 380mg morphine. She called me almost every day, crying on the phone, complaining of terrible distress.

She came to my office, screaming, sobbing, "I can't do this anymore. I can't go down to 380mg morphine a day. I prayed and prayed and prayed but it did not work. I prayed to God to tell you to give me back my medicine."

The change of 400mg to 380mg morphine was a small one, given the large total amount of medication that she was taking. I was not convinced that she was having any physiological difficulty making the change. I believed it was a psychological factor and the anxiety of medication dosage change that were preventing Liz from continuing with her medication reduction.

With the recent success stories of several of my other patients weaning down and even off narcotics, I was confident that Liz could manage with less. Furthermore, if her God told her to come to me, her God must have agreed with my plans.

I denied Liz's request to go back to 400mg morphine. What I did not realize was that, by doing so, I had denied myself an orderly and efficient flow in my office in the immediate future. Liz was no longer satisfied with calling me daily and waiting for my call back. Dragging her body, riddled with terrible degeneration, she took the trouble to come to my office, at least once a week, without an appointment.

Out of respect for her effort, I felt obligated to give her my time to listen to her argument, again and again, regarding her medications. She was not shy about taking up other patients' appointment time. Her presence would be elevated to yet another level, with the endless flow of her tears, dramatic wailing, and feverish preaching about her spirituality.

Finally, the man upstairs answered Liz's prayers.

I gave in.

How much effect would this 20mg morphine difference make on Liz's overall heath? I was not sure how to measure it. How much effect had this 20mg morphine difference made on my physical, psychological, and professional wellbeing? Definitely more than what I had bargained for.

I had to pick my battles.

I agreed to keep Liz on the same amount of medication until her surgery, only if she promised that she would wean down her morphine promptly after her recovery.

Liz was happy. She vowed that she would be very motivated to cut back her medications after her spine surgery. I was not quite as optimistic. I had seen many patients who needed an increased amount of drugs for acute postoperative pain. When they recovered from surgery, trying to wean down their medication was no less than an uphill battle.

Yasmin Hurd, director of the Addiction Institute at Mount Sinai Hospital in New York City, had found that when someone is addicted to opioids, they are often described as having a brain disease. Within the prefrontal cortex of the brain, Hurd found damage to the glutamatergic system, which makes it difficult for neural signals to be transmitted. This is an area of the brain responsible for judgment, decision-making, learning, and memory retention.

Hurd indicated that when an individual's brain is "fundamentally changed" and diseased in this manner, they lose the ability to regulate opioid consumption, unable to quit despite their best efforts—unable to "just say no."[6]

With years of high dosage of opioid consumption, I worried what the prefrontal cortex of Liz's brain would look like.

Two months later, Liz had the extensive corrective spine surgery she needed and came back to me four weeks following her hospital discharge. Liz was, for once in our relationship, in good spirits. She was taking a total of 800mg morphine equivalent pain medication, twice as much as what she was taking before surgery. This indicated that she had a not-so-easy postoperative management process and had to take much more pain medications after her surgery, just as I had predicted and feared.

Liz was in a hard lumbar brace, moving slowly and gingerly, obviously still recovering from surgery. It sometimes takes three to six months or even longer for patients to fully recover from extensive surgeries of this type.

Before I had to chance to start my lecture on how I could only keep up with this new amount of medication for a truly short time before I had to start reducing, Liz asked if she could begin to wean down the narcotics.

"I am ready to cut back," she said. "I feel good. Even it still hurts from the surgery itself, my usual pain from the scoliosis is much better."

My eyes were wide after I heard what she said. I looked out of the window. It was a sunny day. Other than the bright sun, I could not see any stars. But I was sure all the stars were aligned perfectly that day.

Over the next few months, we dramatically tapered the morphine dosage down to a fraction of what Liz had been taking. Although she continued to have subsequent pain, she took the minimal amount of the opioids I prescribed. Liz had a radical change in her behavior. Instead of dreading her appearance in the office like before, I almost looked forward to seeing how much progress Liz had made in the past month. There was no more drama. Liz would talk to me about her art, her family, her new experiments in yoga, and her gym routine.

I was enormously proud of what Liz had done for herself. I often stopped to marvel at what a drastic turn her situation had taken. I would recall the large amount of morphine that Liz required and cringe at the struggles I had with her, trying to reduce her medications. I believed that our success in her pre-surgical opioid reduction had made her post-surgical pain management better.

I still asked myself though: Was I too aggressive toward her narcotic reduction plan before her surgery? Why did she require seemingly much more medication than my other patients? How could I balance individuality and the medical society or government issued guidelines?

Nobody had a good answer for me. "Crossing the river by touching the stones." I would use the wisdom of this ancient Chinese folk saying, to keep learning and adjusting to the needs of my patients, carefully, steadily, but surly.

Paul's Tale of Trouble

PAUL CAME TO my office one afternoon during a raging snowstorm. I didn't expect many patients would come in this kind of weather. Few arrived, but Paul came in on time.

"I have a terrible backache and pain down both of my thighs that hasn't gone away for the past three months," he said to me with desperation in his eyes. "Please, figure out what's wrong and get rid of it."

Paul was a tall, slender man who had worked in construction through his adulthood. Even though he had been taking some time off from his job due to health-related issues, the rest time wasn't making his back pain go away.

"I soak in the tub, put Capsaicin cream on where it hurts, take Advil and muscle relaxants. I go to the gym and exercise, but nothing helps," he said.

"I need stronger pills, Doc. I tried everything under the sun. The only things that have helped me so far are the oxycodone pills.

"I have a wife and two kids to feed, and I need to work. In this condition, I can't do a thing. I have to find a way to get back to work. The boss understands, but there is only so much time he can spare me. I know the pills aren't good for me. I'll try any other treatment you can give me, but I need to be able to function."

By the time Paul came to my office, his pain had been severe and persistent, for several months. It was not responding to conservative treatments, such as NSAIDS, hot compresses and home exercises. I suggested that he start a course of physical therapy.

"Doc, are you kidding me? I can't do physical therapy! That's for people with money and time. And I have neither. I need to work every day. I have no options."

I couldn't argue with him. A good percentage of my patients consist of blue-collar workers. They, like Paul, have to work backbreaking jobs, day in and day out. Years of wear and tear puts a toll on their bodies, not to mention what it does to their minds. Most of their joints are riddled with arthritis. Constant lifting of heavy objects puts them at much higher risk of developing disc herniation of the spine in the neck and low back. Aches and pains are just part of their lives that they have to deal with and accept.

The American College of Physicians treatment guidelines, published in February 2017, highlighted a multitude of choices that don't involve medication. Options such as heat compresses, massage, acupuncture, or spinal manipulation were suggested. Yoga, physical therapy, and chiropractic treatments all look promising and reasonable.

However, in reality, these choices are a luxury, most commonly because they are time consuming and aren't covered by insurance. For example, even if physical therapy, is covered by insurance, patients can only go for a limited number of sessions before insurance coverage runs out.

As a medical provider, I try to always review all treatment modalities which my patients should try and do. However, in reality, I cannot force patients to take time off from their work, stop making money for their families, and start paying out of their pockets to try different things that do not guarantee results.

In this fast-paced day and age, nobody has the time to let their aches and pains heal on their own. Everyone wants a miracle that instantly takes all their troubles away.

For Paul, it was out of the question that he would be willing to try a few weeks of physical therapy. We needed to get him back working and functioning again, fast.

Paul's physical examination showed moderate to severe lumbar spinal nerve root irritation. I decided to send him for a lumbar spine MRI to evaluate his spinal discs. Fortunately for Paul, the radiology services at the hospital near my office had a lot of cancellations that day and we could slip Paul in for an immediate exam of his lumbar spine.

The MRI showed that Paul had developed two large lumbar disc herniations in his spine at the level of L2/3 and L3/4, impinging on his L3, L4 nerves. It explained why he had excruciating pain in his low back and the front of his thighs and legs. His pain was real and acute. I understood why he made such an effort to get to me on that day.

For pain associated with nerve impingement that is not responding to conservative treatments, the next step is a lumbar epidural steroid injection to deliver the anti-inflammatory medication directly to the site of the problem.

Paul broke out in a sweat when I told him about his injury. He requested that the injection to be done as soon as possible, because he wanted to feel better in order to get back to his regular work schedule.

I took him into the procedure suite and positioned him on his stomach. Under X-ray guidance, I performed an epidural steroid injection at the level where his irritated nerves were located. Immediately after I had completed the injection, Paul turned over and sat up. I asked him how he felt, and he looked at me in amazement.

"I feel fine," he said and grinned broadly. "My back and legs already are feeling better."

The mixture that I injected into Paul's back contained some lidocaine, in addition to cortisone. Lidocaine was the numbing agent that works in minutes, as it was placed in the correct spot, further confirming our diagnosis of pain from his herniated discs. That was why Paul was already feeling better.

However, lidocaine wears off in a few hours. Paul would likely feel his pain again later that day. In the next two to five days, the cortisone would "kick in" and hopefully offer long-lasting relief. If the pain were still severe, he could receive another injection in a month or so. The injection diagnosed the problem, and treated it as well, but it was not a cure at all.

"What? It takes two to five days to work. And I may need more injections to feel better?" Paul yelled out when he heard my instructions before leaving.

"That isn't going to work for me. I have to go back to work tomorrow. How am I going to do that? Doc? You've got to give me something better so I can handle my job. I really need a few of those oxycodone pills. I promise you that I won't use it for anything else but to help me get through the day. The oxycodone was the only thing that helped me in the past three months."

I was really reluctant to give Paul any opioids such as oxycodone because they would not treat the root of the problem; they would just numb the brain not to think about the pain. Worse yet, the human body gets used to the medication and patients usually need more opioids to achieve the same effect with long-term use.

In Paul's case, he did have severe pain. The cause was obvious, and his agony was intense, despite the treatment. He did have to hold a full-time construction job. Constant pain would make his workdays intolerable without effective medication. The situation did not seem to leave any other options for him, or for me.

I asked Paul to sit down while I went over the dangers of opioid use. We agreed that as soon as his pain decreased, we would wean him off.

A month later, Paul showed up for his follow-up appointment on time, accompanied by his wife, Susan.

"She wanted to thank you for making me much easier to live with," he said, as Susan gave me an unexpected hug. Paul told me that he still experienced episodes of pain, but nothing like what he had gone through before.

"I got to hand it to you, Doc. You sure knew how to deal with my terrible back. But I still have bad days. On those days, I definitely need my oxycodone to get me through."

That's when Paul rejected my plan to wean him off oxycodone. I insisted that since his back pain was better, he needed to start cutting down on the pills to get through his days. I scheduled him for another epidural injection, hoping his pain would eventually decrease to a point where he would not need any opioids to tolerate his workdays.

Over the next year or so, Paul's pain was up and down. He did have months that he didn't need to take any opioids when his back was in remission. He also had episodes of relapse and had to fall back to oxycodone to work full time.

This pattern is rather common among my patients. Disc herniation, like other chronic back pain conditions, may never heal completely. Patients are vulnerable and they may suffer flare ups of severe pain. Sometimes the nerve irritation rises from known events, such as lifting a heavy object, a car accident, or a fall. Sometimes, an inciting event cannot be identified. It just happens. Patients can wake up with severe pain. Or pain can come on while they sit at the dinner table. It can be rather frustrating for them.

"In order to stay away from me, your pain management doctor," I tell every one of my patients, "you need to maintain a healthy weight, do your core strengthening exercises every day, and avoid doing things that can hurt you, such as lifting heavy items."

Paul continued to work in construction. How could he possibly stay away from strenuous activities which constantly put stress on his spine? Having flare ups was just a matter of frequency for him.

During this period of time, Paul's wife also became my patient. She worked as a waitress and had to lift heavy trays full of food, plates, and glassware, all day long. She had her share of chronic low back pain and needed spinal treatment as well.

Paul brought Susan along for her first appointment as a patient when he had a follow-up visit with me. I first took Paul's chart and talked with him. After we were done, I picked up Susan's chart, and got ready to talk with her.

When I glanced at the charts, to my surprise, the dates of birth on both charts were the same. I thought it must have been an error made by the front desk staff. When they created Susan's chart, they apparently used her husband's information as a template. They changed the name but forgot to change the birthday.

"I am terribly sorry, Susan, but my staff put your husband's birthday on your chart. What an embarrassing mistake. What is your birthday?" I apologized to Susan and Paul and was ready to make corrections on the chart.

"That is my correct birthday. We have the same birthday," Susan said as she laughed and grabbed her husband's hand. Her eyes grew bright and happy.

"Guess what? I have a twin sister. And listen to this: She married a guy with the exact same birthday as ours."

I almost fell off the chair in amazement. What was the chance of that happening?

Needless to say, Susan and Paul made such an impression on me. However, what made them a memorable couple was that they were always sweet and happy to be together when they came to my office. They would talk to me about their two beautiful children—a boy and a girl—their work and their parents.

Before long, Paul's sister, Erin, and his parents all became my patients for low back pain. I could see where Paul's bad back came from. In addition to his back-breaking job, he also inherited it and was probably born with weak spinal structures.

Susan was also getting epidural injections for her lumbar spine problem, from time to time. She would thank me profusely after each treatment. "I hate to take any medication. These injections do ease my pain and allow me to work and play with my children."

Our relationship went on an even course for two more years. On another wintry day, Paul returned to my office after he had shoveled snow, following a big storm. From all that work, he developed severe pain in his back and right leg the very next day. Only this time around, he had pain in the back of his left leg, which was new. His left foot was so weak that he limped and dragged his foot while walking.

His left ankle reflexes were absent on examination, along with significant weakness in his left foot. I immediately sent him to get a new MRI and referred him to a spine surgeon. Paul's weakness in his left leg was a sign of severe nerve root compression. The MRI confirmed a new large, herniated disc at L5/S1 level, pressing on his nerve roots. He had no choice but to undergo lumbar spine surgery.

Paul shook his head. He then he began to cry in the office. Susan became terribly concerned about him and the impending surgery.

"We don't have a choice this time, Paul," I explained. "I wish we could make it better in some other way, but you need the surgery to avoid things becoming worse, such as permanent weakness in your legs and irreversible damage to your nerves."

He nodded, wiped his eyes, and blew his nose. "I'll have to get through it, and I have a lot of people who care about me. I'll be okay."

And he was. Paul's surgery was successful. He healed well and gained back all his strength in his left foot. However, he complained of pain in his low back and numbness in his left leg that persisted. At first, I provided Paul with oxycodone, as he recovered from his surgical pain. We agreed to wean him off within two months after surgery, when he healed.

In two months, the time came to wean him off the oxycodone. Paul pleaded with me. "I still have terrible pain in my back, and I just returned to work. There is no way I can survive, day to day without the pills."

I contacted his surgeon and discussed Paul's case with him at length. Apparently, all the test results and MRIs showed that Paul was on the correct course of recovery. My question was: Did Paul have a real reason for his continued use of oxycodone?

Everybody's experience of pain and recovery after surgery is different. Sometimes, it takes longer for patients to recover. Therefore, it was reasonable that Paul still needed pain medication for another month or so because he likely was still in recovery.

To make things even more complicated, some patients are never free of pain after major spine surgery. This chronic persistent pain is known as "post laminectomy pain syndrome." Was Paul developing this chronic syndrome and if so, how long should he need to be kept on opioids? These were difficult questions for me or any doctors to answer.

My next plan was to aggressively use non-opioid options to treat Paul's pain. We tried neuropathic agents, which are medications for nerve pain, such as Lyrica and gabapentin, medications used along with the oxycodone. Then I prescribed physical therapy, acupuncture, and massage, which Paul finally agreed to do this time around.

We also tried different steroid injections to the spine. I did frequent urine toxicology screening to closely monitor Paul's opioid use.

Almost a year went by after Paul's low back surgery, Paul's toxicology tests always came back with appropriate results. On the other hand, his pain never seemed to subside, despite all the effort and treatment. He became a regular who would come for his monthly oxycodone refills, but he became less talkative and quite morose, although he denied being depressed.

When he talked, he would complain that the pain medication that I gave him was not enough. He had to reduce his workdays, due to his suffering. I hardly saw Susan or Paul's family in my office any longer. I didn't like the way things appeared with Paul. I could not put my finger on it, but I knew it was time to discuss weaning off narcotics with him and a host of other issues.

Paul was reluctant but he did not make much fuss. I gave him a weaning schedule for his pain medication. We agreed on a plan to slowly taper off his oxycodone over the course of two months.

Paul didn't show up for his follow-up appointment the next month, which was a signal that something might have gone wrong. I left a message for him to call, but nobody called back.

Two months passed but there was still no response from him, despite repeated efforts by our office team to reach him.

"Maybe he was able to wean himself off the oxycodone and did not need to come see me for any more prescription refills," I thought with optimism.

Three months went by before Paul and Susan showed up at my office together, for Paul's appointment.

Susan got right to the point. "Paul and I are here together, trying to start our lives over again. We need your help. Paul has been abusing oxycodone."

It was one thing for me to suspect something was going on. It was still a big shock for me to have my suspicions confirmed. How? How did Paul manage to be a drug abuser and stay off my radar?

He was on a low dose regimen and was never early for his medication refills. He never had a dirty urine sample. The drug monitoring system, I STOP, never showed that he received narcotics from other providers. He had real pain due to his spine and needed the medication. He was actively involved in non-narcotic treatments to improve his life. He had a job and he worked. He had a loving family who offered a good social support system. He simply did not fit the profile.

It turned out that Paul complained of persistent pain ever since his low back surgery. When he took his oxycodone, the medication only took the edge off his symptoms. In search of better pain relief, he had gone online and learned that if he snorted oxycodone, it would work better. He tried it, and before long, he became addicted to the euphoria associated with the process.

Paul started using oxycodone for pleasure instead of pain control. In order not to leave any trail or records on the I STOP, Paul would avoid going to other doctors for prescriptions. He purchased more oxycodone on the street. He was also careful not to use other illicit substances or any other prescriptional opioids, in order to have appropriate results on his urine toxicology screening tests.

"Okay. I'm ready to come clean about abusing drugs," Paul sighed, "but I still have pain and I don't know what to do."

I thanked both Paul and Susan for their trust in me to tell me about Paul's drug problem. I explained to them that he needed to be admitted for in patient detox. I would continue to do my best to find a way to control his pain. His options, however, can not include any opioids. We all agreed with the plan.

"He's a good dad," Susan said softly. "Our kids don't know everything yet, but they know Daddy is sick and needs help. Our whole family will deal with this together."

I spent the rest of the day seeing patients but could not stop thinking about Paul and Susan. It was troubling to learn about Paul's trouble with drugs. I wondered what to expect concerning Paul's future and that of his family, as I feared more difficulty ahead.

A week later, I was told that Paul entered a detox center, where he did become clean of oxycodone. He was then under the care of an addiction psychiatrist who prescribed Suboxone, a medication that is crafted to relieve the craving for drugs. I treated him for his condition with steroid injections several times during the next two years.

Then he stopped coming to see me altogether.

I thought of Paul and Susan often, hoping that the reason for his absence was because his pain was under control and his life was in good order.

Another two years went by, when I started periodically seeing his sister, Erin, again for her pain-related condition. Erin told me that she had not seen Paul for at least a year. She would cry every time she mentioned Paul. She missed him, but he would not see any of his family.

Over the grapevine, Erin had heard that Paul wasn't doing well. He was in and out of rehab and was unable to completely stay away from drugs. Paul was slowly sinking, and Susan had no choice but to take the children and leave.

My heart ached for Susan, Paul, and their extended family.

A few months after I learned about Paul's situation, Susan came back to my office for treatment for her low back pain. She told me that she and Paul had sought a divorce because life together was just too hard for them, and for the kids.

Then, with time, both Paul and Susan started dating other people and found new lives. The two kids lived with Susan but had visitations with Paul. All the adults and kids seemed to get along simply fine. Things seemed to have turned the corner and were on an upswing. Susan started to laugh again and shared her work and family whereabouts when she came, just like before. I was relieved and incredibly happy for her and all of them.

When the news came in that Paul died, it was unexpected. And then again, maybe not so much. Erin brought the news with her when she came for a treatment. Paul's girlfriend told Erin that Paul had died in his sleep from an apparent heart attack.

"How could he have had a heart attack at age forty-four?" I asked with true candor. His sister was silent.

When I saw Susan from time to time, the tears didn't stop when she recalled all that she had been through with Paul. She told me that the two children were in the house with Paul the night he died. Both of them had developed post-traumatic stress disorder and had problems in school. Susan was working hard and raising them, while trying to get them back on track, as much as she could.

Paul's parents, after all these years, came back to see me for their chronic spine treatments. Paul's mother was a petite, but strong woman. She seemed upbeat all the time. I avoided talking to her about anything other than her own spinal issues.

One day, without any warning, she sighed and said, "The pain in my spine is not my biggest problem. The pain in my heart is my real issue." She broke down crying. "You know that I lost my son to drugs. But I also lost my two grandchildren too. We now live in the house where they used to live. Paul's two children will not visit us in our place because it reminds them of their dad. They don't want to have anything to do with us and won't even talk to us on the phone. We have not seen our grandchildren for years and I miss them so much."

Paul was the one who used and abused drugs. He had destroyed his life. He had also scarred the entire family: Susan, Erin, his parents, and especially his children.

Almost ten years have passed since I first met Paul. To this day, I often think about him and his family. I can still clearly visualize that moment when Susan and Paul were laughing at my surprise with their birthday facts; when they came to confess the drug abuse; when Erin told me about Paul's death; and when Paul's mom broke down and cried her heart out in my office.

I can't help but wonder what I would have done differently if I had just met Paul today? If I never had given him the oxycodone, would his life be different? Would it be realistic to deny a patient in acute and severe pain all opioids? If he had been given more oxycodone, would that have prevented him from finding "better" ways for pain control online and resorting to snorting drugs?

I probably will never stop thinking and wondering.

The Drug That Killed Prince

FENTANYL IS AN extremely potent drug at the center of the new overdose epidemic and is presenting unique challenges for law enforcement officials, healthcare professionals, and society as a whole, because it's so deadly, versatile, and profitable.

Between April of 2020 to April 2021, according to data released from the Center of Disease Control's National Center for Health Statistics, over 100,000 Americans died of drug overdose as the COVID pandemic continued to spread nationwide, surpassing the toll of gun violence and car accidents combined. The rise in deaths was mainly fueled by widespread use of fentanyl, a fast-acting drug that is fifty to one hundred times more powerful than morphine[7].

The raw material of fentanyl is mainly produced in China. Mexican drug cartels, who mix fentanyl with heroin and other substances and then smuggle those mixtures across the U.S.-Mexico border. It is being trafficked with vast dealer networks and by small-time operators ordering the narcotics online, according to Ben Westhoff, the author of Fentanyl, Inc. How Rogue Chemists Created the Deadliest Wave of the Opioid Epidemic.

The amount of fentanyl coming into the U.S. via the mail system is growing—in smaller packages and at much greater potency. Fentanyl is easier and cheaper to produce than heroin, which is derived from poppy plants. With fentanyl, there are no crops, just chemicals.

"You can make it as strong as you want, in bulk and very fast," Tim Reagan, a Cincinnati-based DEA agent, said. And because it's so potent, a little bit goes a long way, making it extremely profitable.[8]

"Fentanyl is everywhere," Barbara Carreno said, a spokeswoman for the federal Drug Enforcement Agency[9]

A main reason that fentanyl has become a popular street drug is that it is not only more potent than heroin, but also far cheaper. Addiction Resource.

---

7   https://www.nytimes.com/2021/11/17/health/drug-overdoses-fentanyl-deaths.html
8   https://www.advantagebhs.org/news.cms/2017/135/
9   https://www.usatoday.com/story/news/nation/2017/08/31/fentanyl-opioid-fueling-new-overdose-crisis/616826001/

net [10]lists that a single dose of fentanyl is considered to be 100 mcg-400 mcg and will cost about two dollars or less. Each dose of Heroin, cocaine, or MDMA will cost twenty dollars. When anyone compares the average cost of a single dose of each of the street drugs, it is easy to see why fentanyl makes a cheap substitute or filler.

But what does this "street drug" have to do with my practice?

Fentanyl is widely used in the medical field. There are three main forms doctors use. One is the intravenous form which is often used for relief of severe acute pain during and immediately after surgery. Because of its high potency and risk of slowing down patient's breathing, patients receiving intravenous fentanyl require special and constant monitoring by doctors or nurses in the hospital. It is not even allowed to be used on regular patient wards. Only special locations caring for patients with acute and severe pain such as the operating room, post anesthesia care unit, and the intensive care unit have permission for administering intravenous fentanyl.

The other main form of fentanyl for medical use is a transdermal patch. Fentanyl patches are used to relieve severe chronic pain in people who are expected to need pain medication around the clock. Transdermal Fentanyl is applied to the skin once approximately every seventy-two hours.

After a fentanyl patch is applied, the medication passes into the skin a little at a time. Patients may take up to twenty-four hours to feel the full effect of the patch. For the same reason, the medication can stay in the body for days after the patch is removed. It is only used for patients who have already been taking other narcotics on a regular basis. Like any other opioids, with proper use, fentanyl patch can be a good treatment option for some patients. For example, because it is passed through skin, patients with difficulty swallowing or with painful mouth or gastrointestinal tract diseases can bypass the need to swallow pain pills. Furthermore, because the patch only needs to be changed every seventy-two hours, it can be advantageous for patients who are unable to remember their medication intake schedule. It is less labor intensive for caretakers to help manage fentanyl patch.

The third form of fentanyl is a trans mucosal form such as Actiq which is a fentanyl lollipop, or Fentora which is a tablet. Both of them dissolve in the mouth for absorption across the buccal mucosa. It gets absorbed by the body and acts quickly. This form of fentanyl is only FDA approved for the treatment of acute and severe pain associated with cancer. They allow patients to control their terrible pain at home without the need of an intravenous line or being in the hospital. As for all fentanyl products, patients need to be opioid tolerant, meaning have already been taking other opioids on a long term and regular basis before they can be given trans mucosal fentanyl.

10   https://www.addictionresource.net

One can imagine how intravenous and trans mucosal forms of fentanyl can easily be used for recreational purposes because they are very fast acting. When I first learned about the transdermal form of fentanyl, I regarded it as one of the safest methods to treat patients who needed opioids. I found myself dead wrong during my pain management fellowship. One of my professors was sued because his patient whom he gave fentanyl patch prescriptions was found dead, overdosed from fentanyl. I could not comprehend how people can get high from a patch that takes days to release the active ingredient.

The methods in which fentanyl patch is used to get high are quite creative and ingenious. According to the article on the Recovery Village website[11], "Fentanyl patch abuse is possible . . . when someone removes the gel from the patch and injects it. The person may take the gel, heat it, or mix it with water and then use a needle to inject it into their vein." Furthermore, "Fentanyl patch abuse can occur when someone chews the patches and then the drug is absorbed by the mucous membranes, or when they smoke the gel that's inside, or when they steep the fentanyl patches in hot water and drink the liquid as if it's tea."

I cannot help but wonder what great inventions and discoveries the world might have if these people put their minds and energy into the right endeavor.

For the past decade or so, pain management specialists like me have refrained from prescribing trans mucosal fentanyl, except on rare occasions and for specific needs, such as acute and severe cancer pain. For transdermal fentanyl patches, patients need to be carefully selected with thorough education regarding the correct way to use them. I have a handful of patients using them.

However, fentanyl found other ways to grab my attention.

Sarah has been my long-term patient for her chronic neck pain. She came in one day for a follow up appointment. Her eyes were red. Her face was swollen. She slumped in the chair and started sobbing when I asked what happened to her.

"My grandson died. He went to a party and never came back. He overdosed on fentanyl. That's what the police told us." Sarah tried to wipe away her tears, "his friend died too. Two kids. Gone. Just like that. I am sure he did not know what he was taking at the party."

This was not the first time my patients recounted someone they knew died from fentanyl overdose. The victims were typically young adults. It would not be known if my patient's grandson knew what he was taking. However, more and more overdose deaths are related to use of fentanyl involvement without the knowledge of drug users.

On November 20th, 2021, the New York Times published an article by Sarah Maslin Nir, entitled, "Inside Fentanyl's Mounting Death Toll: 'This

11   https://www.therecoveryvillage.com

is Poison.'" The article reports that, "It (Fentanyl) is spliced into party drugs where it can be consumed unwittingly."[12] In the summer of 2021 on Long Island, six people were killed by a single batch of fentanyl laced cocaine. Sarah Maslin Nir calls fentanyl "the third wave of the opioid epidemic that began in the 1990s with prescription pills, followed by exploding heroin use."

One of the reasons that fentanyl has become so deadly, Ms. Nir points out, is because drug dealers would mix fentanyl into cocaine, heroin, or marijuana. Since there is no quality control, people may mix in more fentanyl in batches that already contain fentanyl, making it extra lethal. People who already developed high tolerance to cocaine and heroin may still be new to fentanyl, making their bodies highly susceptible to the fatal effect of this synthetic opioid.

According to the article, "In New York City, the majority of autopsies of overdose deaths now reveal that fentanyl was involved, including that of actor Michael K. Williams, found dead in his Brooklyn apartment."

The opioid addiction crisis gripping the nation has been bad enough, but now drug officials and first responders increasingly see overdose cases of heroin, cocaine, or prescription drugs mixed with Fentanyl.

Other than clamping down on drug trafficking and increasing in rehabilitation programs, and education on drug abstinence, the availability of naloxone is essential to save lives.

Singer and entertainer, Demi Lovato, almost died in July 2018, from a mixture containing fentanyl, and was saved by an injection of naloxone—a drug that can bring life back to those who are on the edge of death from narcotic overdose.

Naloxone is an antagonist of the opioid receptors, meaning it can block the receptors and reverse the effect of opioids. Naloxone can be used as a nose spray, or an injection into the muscles or veins. It can then reverse the effects of opioids, including extreme drowsiness, slowed breathing, or loss of consciousness, therefore restoring breathing and saving people's lives.

In "Review of naloxone safety for opioid overdose,"[13] D.P. Werbeling set out to evaluate interventions to improve opioid prescribing practices, including the co-prescription of naloxone.

It was found that giving this drug to patients on opioid therapy for chronic pain was associated with fewer opioid-related emergency department visits, especially among patients receiving high doses of prescription opioids.

---

12   https://www.nytimes.com/2021/11/20/nyregion/fentanyl-opioid-deaths.html

13   Wermeling, D.P., Review of naloxone safety for opioid overdose: practical considerations for new technology and expanded public access Therapeutic Advances in Drug Safety, 2015. 6(1): p. 20-31.

Studies as such help doctors like me to understand when to provide selected high-risk patients with a Naloxone prescription.

Physicians may not be able to prevent illegal production or street sale of fentanyl, but we can keep the prescription form of fentanyl out of the wrong hands with careful medication prescribing and patient educations. We can also provide the lifesaving naloxone to high-risk patients to minimize risk of opioid overdose.

"Cannabis is the single most versatile remedy
and the most useful plant on Earth."
— Ethan Russo, M.D.

Cannabis, Medical Marijuana

IN JULY 2014, the governor signed the Compassionate Care Act into law, legalizing medical marijuana in New York State. Participation in the program was limited to people with a handful of serious conditions—including cancer, HIV or AIDS, amyotrophic lateral sclerosis (ALS), Parkinson's disease, multiple sclerosis, spinal cord injury with spasticity, epilepsy, inflammatory bowel disease, neuropathy, and Huntington's Disease—and thus excluded many individuals who otherwise might benefit from it.

Qualified patients are not able to receive medical marijuana from a designated dispensary unless they are registered with the state. At the time of registration, the state Health Department will issue patients registry identification cards. In order to get a card, patients must first be certified by a healthcare provider. The doctor or nurse practitioner must also register with the state and have completed a four-hour training course.

I did not pay much attention to this law being passed at the time, because majority of my patients would be excluded from the program. My only encounter with marijuana at the time the law was passed was a day as a college student, when I smelled something unusual in the air.

"That's marijuana," a friend of mine told me. The aroma was so distinctive; it made a lasting impression on me. I had no interest in getting to know about the plant. I was sure that it was an intoxicating substance, a gateway drug. Any illicit substance is poison, I reminded myself; something to stay away from. That was the belief I never expected to change.

Then, I met Sam, who was a retired schoolteacher in his sixties. He had a brain tumor and underwent craniotomy surgery twice to remove the cancer. The tumor and surgeries had left him a crater the size of a deck of playing cards, on his right skull. He also had to have his right eye removed.

Although one would not be able to tell by just looking at him. His prosthetic eye was so beautifully made; it looked just like his own. His chestnut-colored hair grew back dark and thick after his chemotherapy. They had perfectly covered the crater on the skull. However, his almost perfect look did not help the fact that there was still a small amount of cancer left in his brain. The small part was deemed too risky to be removed.

His cancer continued to give him severe pain in his skull, right eye socket, and sinuses. The pain waxed and waned depending on the tumor growth and his radiation treatment cycles. I provided Sam with monthly prescription of oxycodone for pain control.

Sam was careful with his medications. He would take no pills on a good day and only used them as needed. After two years of being relatively stable with pain and his cancer, Sam had a bad flare up. Pain became persistent and severe despite his cancer treatment. I had to increase his daily dosage again and again, in a short period of time.

When he reached the amount of oxycodone 20mg, twenty pills a day, I got very worried. It is known that cancer patients sometimes require a large amount of opioids due to their disease progression. However, I was getting uncomfortable with where things were going. Soon, Sam could have intolerable side effects if we had to keep raising the dosage. And his body may develop tolerance to narcotics to make his pain management even more challenging.

At that time, I heard about a local physician who just returned to the area from California. The doctor had more than a decade of experience prescribing medical marijuana to patients for various diseases, including cancer. I sent Sam to her.

"Sam, you got nothing to lose. Just try it. Maybe it would work along with the oxycodone, and it may help manage your pain."

"Dr. Shue, is medical marijuana the same as the CBD being sold online and in drug stores? How come I need to see a doctor to get it. Can I just buy them off the shelf or online, on my own?" Sam asked.

Sam's confusion is very common. With CBD products gaining popularity, they are seen in almost every health food store and on pharmacy shelf.

"Those CBD products sold over the counter and online are made from hemp, a relative of marijuana. It is considered less potent than CBD from marijuana. These products are not regulated either. Unless you know a credible source, quality is not guaranteed. For your severe pain problems, it is best to consult with a medical professional before you make any purchase. And medical marijuana has other important ingredients besides CBD, which you cannot get from over-the-counter products," I told Sam.

Sam was finally convinced. Both he and I had become desperate.

One month after he started the medical marijuana program, Sam called my office.

"Dr. Shue, thank you so much for sending me to the marijuana doctor. I am using medical marijuana and it works so well that I weaned myself off the oxycodone. I feel like I can live my life again."

From twenty pills of 20mg oxycodone to zero, in such a short time. With well controlled pain! Is medical marijuana really the miracle drug?

Sam's experience completely changed my view on marijuana. I started paying attention to it as an alternative option for my other patients who suffer from cancer and multiple sclerosis.

At the end of 2016, the New York State Department of Health added "chronic pain" as a qualifying condition for medical marijuana[14]. Because chronic pain is seen in many medical conditions, the product became available to far more people, including most of my patients.

As I started speaking to the people I treat, about the medical marijuana program and sending them to the other medical providers for the certification process, more and more of my patients requested that I become certified as a medical marijuana physician. Who knew, that two decades after my first encounter with it, I would take that four-hour-long class, study, pass my exam, and become an advocate of this useful substance.

In the U.S., medical marijuana—also referred to as medical cannabis—is legal in an expanding number of states. The plant itself, or extract of the plant is carefully processed from the dried leaves and buds of the cannabis plant. It can be used for pain, nausea, and side effects of medical treatments. Depending on why a person is using the drug, treatment may be short term or continue for years.

Many people, including certain celebrities, have vouched for the effectiveness of medicinal use of marijuana.

Actor Sir Patrick Stewart recently discussed his use of marijuana on a daily basis to combat his arthritic symptoms. He's not alone. Actress and talk show host, Whoopi Goldberg, has used it routinely for medical issues that plague her, such as sciatica. In agreement with its usage because of personal physical issues are Lady Gaga and Melissa Ethridge among many others.

The award-winning actor Stewart shone a light on his regimen when he endorsed the United Kingdom's program aimed at exploring the benefits of cannabis-based medicines.

Stewart, who suffers from severe arthritis, referred to the cannabinoid biomedicine program out of Oxford University as "an important step forward for Britain in a field of research that has for too long been held back by prejudice, fear, and ignorance."[15]

"Several years ago, I was examined by a doctor in Los Angeles and given a prescription which gave me legal permission to purchase several types of

14   https://spectrumlocalnews.com/nys/buffalo/news/2016/12/1/
doh-chronic-pain-new-york-medical-marijuana-program
15   https://www.hollywoodreporter.com/news/general-news/patrick-
stewart-reveals-medical-marijuana-use-arthritis-986885/

cannabis-based products from a registered outlet. I was advised they might help the crippling osteoarthritis in both of my hands," Stewart said. Medical marijuana has been helping him ever since and he "regularly purchase(s) an ointment, spray, and edibles."

According to the Disease Control and Prevention Program in 2020, over 24 percent of adults in the U.S.—or 54.4 million people—have been diagnosed with osteoarthritis. Of that number, 43.5 percent were found to suffer limitations in movement. Stewart shared that his arthritis is believed to be genetic as his mother, he recalled, "had badly distorted and painful hands."

"I believe that the ointment and spray have significantly reduced the stiffness and pain in my own hands. I can now make fists, which was not the case for a long while before I began this treatment," he said.

There are many individuals and groups who oppose the use of marijuana for countless reasons and concerns. An honest and open discussion must be brought to the public from all sides of the spectrum.

For some physicians, medical marijuana represents an uncomfortable territory to tread. Unlike other medication that we use, medical marijuana has not undergone rigorous clinical studies or trials. If a physician is to prescribe it, just like any other medication for patients, the substance needs to be studied and put through trials, approved by the FDA, before we prescribe uniformly like any other medication.

Once upon a time, the medical community thought, as I did, that treating with opioids was wholly appropriate. It took us decades to realize that the inappropriate use of opioids had resulted in the opioid crisis and numerous fatalities. Would similar disastrous results ensure if we start widely using medical marijuana before further research is done?

Despite all the testing and furor over medical marijuana, the FDA has not approved the drug for use as a safe and effective drug for any indication, except for one product—Epidiolex.

By June 2018, The U.S. Food and Drug Administration approved Epidiolex (cannabidiol) oral solution for the treatment of seizures associated with two rare and severe forms of epilepsy, called Lennox-Gastaut syndrome and Dravet syndrome. This is the first FDA-approved drug that contains a purified drug substance derived from marijuana.[16]

The agency has also approved two drugs—Dronabinol and nabilone—which are used to treat nausea and boost appetite, for cancer and AIDS patients. These two drugs contain a synthetic version of substances that are present in the marijuana plant, and supposedly act similarly marijuana. However, from my anecdotal observation, these two drugs are off limited use

---

16   https://www.epilepsy.com/treatment/alternative-therapies/medical-marijuana#:

due to lack of insurance coverage or effectiveness. "They just did not work the same like marijuana." one patient told me.

The FDA's role in the regulation of drugs, including marijuana and marijuana-derived products, focuses on a review of applications to market drugs to determine if they are safe and effective for their intended indications. The FDA's drug approval process requires well designed clinical trials to provide the agency with the scientific data for its approval decisions.

Without the necessary clinical trials and data, the FDA cannot determine if a drug is safe and effective. For certain drugs, such as marijuana, the lack of FDA approval and regulation means that the purity and potency of the drug may not be consistent. It may take years for these research and reviews to complete to prove that the cannabinoid products are indicated for a variety of medical conditions.

The federal government has been involved in facilitating medical marijuana research. The National Institute on Drug Abuse (NIDA), within the National Institutes of Health, provides research-grade marijuana for scientific study. The agency has contracted with organizations, such as the University of Mississippi to grow marijuana for research purposes. At these appointed facilities, marijuana of varying potencies and compositions is being cultivated and researched.

A large number of states have either passed laws that remove restrictions on the medical use of marijuana or are considering doing so. The FDA supports these researchers who conduct important and well-controlled clinical trials which may lead to the development of more safe and effective marijuana products to treat a larger number of medical conditions.

At this point in time, marijuana remains a Schedule One drug under federal law. Therefore, federal law regulating marijuana supersedes state law. This means, in theory, people may still be arrested and charged with possession of an illegal substance under federal law, in states where medical marijuana is legal. This contradiction in legalities places the medical marijuana patients in a rather precarious situation, depending on where he or she lives.

Each state formulates its own rules and regulations regarding medical or recreational marijuana use. The state determines who may use it and how the product is dispensed to patients. Each state has its process for certifying and registering eligible patients. Some have designated dispensaries, or medical marijuana centers, where people can get the product and information on dosing, as well as what form to use for their condition.

While waiting for more scientific and clinical evidence to facilitate FDA approval or change in federal laws, some groups started actively advocating the use of medical marijuana for their members.

In the New York Times article titled "Veterans Groups Push for Medical Marijuana to Treat PTSD," [17] author Reggie Ugwu reports that:

For a long time, the veterans' groups have been working to advocate for medical marijuana use. They argue that access to medical marijuana could ease suffering and reduce suicide rates among soldiers who return from the horrors of war.

In 2016, the American Legion asked Congress to remove the drug from the list of Schedule One narcotics—a class that includes heroin, LSD, and other drugs that have "no accepted medical use" and a high potential for abuse—and reclassify it to a lower schedule grade. It also called on the Drug Enforcement Administration to license more privately funded growers to focus on medical research.

The current classification means that veterans cannot get coverage for medical marijuana, even in the states that have legalized it.

I have heard specific complaints, first-hand, from my veteran patients. Due to the legal status of medical marijuana at a federal level, my patients have to pay out of their own pocket for medical marijuana, which can total two hundred dollars or more a week, depending on how much a patient uses. This creates a significant financial burden on these people who have a fixed monthly income.

Other patients who are federal government employees have to pass on the option of medical marijuana altogether because they would lose their jobs if they were caught using a federally illegal substance.

As more patients come to me for medical marijuana prescriptions, I realize that the information I received from that four-hour course was grossly insufficient. In addition to a limited supply of effective educational programs and scientific journal publications, I found myself having to learn a completely new concept and system on my own for the use of medical marijuana.

For instance, the medical marijuana dispensary works differently from a traditional pharmacy. Since I am not a patient, I am not permitted to go into a dispensary because only a medical marijuana card holder can gain access to it. But new patients interested in the program invariably ask me questions about the process and the pricing in the dispensary.

To learn more about this substance, I ask all my patients to share their experience with me, once they have been to the dispensary and have tried their products. One of them said that going to a local dispensary was like entering a candy store. There are all types of the cannabis products from which to choose. With any other regular medication, the pharmacists and patients would strictly follow the exact dosage and directions from the physician who writes the prescription. For medical marijuana in the state of New York, the physician can provide a general recommendation on the prescription.

There is an option for the physician to give the pharmacist total flexibility stating, "usage per pharmacist's recommendation." The pharmacists at the dispensary then advise patients which product would best fit their pain issues and other concerns, and what they may expect after using the drugs.

Finding the correct type and strength of medical marijuana can be a frustrating process. Like any medication, it can take some trial and error for patients to find a product that suits them best.

In the United States, some dispensaries provide one-stop shopping for edibles, tinctures, salves, sprays, and soft buds to cook or smoke. In the state of New York, there were no whole plant products available initially. However, since around 2021, my patients informed me that whole plant products, such as dried flowers and buds have become available in New York.

Each above form of medical marijuana has a whole spectrum of ratios of the two major cannabinoids found in cannabis plants, which are THC (tetrahydrocannabinol) and CBD (cannabidiol).

THC is the primary active component of cannabis. It is psychoactive which can make people feel "high." CBD is considered to be non-psychoactive. When CBD is used in conjunction with THC, it helps reduce side effects associated with THC, including heart palpitation, paranoia, hunger, and the feeling of "high." Both cannabinoids are believed to have an impressive list of ways they support the human body.

As stated in the book, Chronic Relief by author Nishi Whitely, THC is a strong anti-inflammatory and painkiller. It is also a bronchodilator, anti-spasmodic, muscle relaxant, a powerful neuroprotectant, and antioxidant. In fact, it is believed to have twenty times the anti-inflammatory power of aspirin and twice that of hydrocortisone[18].

On the other hand, CBD is believed to reduce seizure activities, anxiety, and nausea. It also has anti-inflammatory, antioxidant (stronger than vitamins C and E), anti-depressant and anti-psychotic properties.

CBD's combined strong anti-inflammatory, antioxidant and neuro-protective properties can have great promise for the treatment of Alzheimer's, Parkinson's disease, and other neurodegenerative-related diseases. Some doctors think that CBD also helps regulate blood pressure and can reduce the growth of breast cancer and certain other types of cancer cells, while protecting healthy cells.

Scientists believe that cannabis benefits so many different illnesses, because its active pharmacological components mimic an internal chemical system in the human body that keeps our health in balance—the Endocannabinoid System (ECS). This system plays an important role in the regulation of pain,

18   https://mychronicrelief.com/cannabis-book/

memory, mood, immunity, and stress. It is further suggested that anandamide contributes to exercise-induced euphoria, commonly known as "runner's high." That explains why taking medical marijuana, which activates the Endocannabinoid System, can make people feel elated and improve pain and mood.

When patients first come to discuss medical marijuana with me, most of them say, "Can you give me the kind of medical marijuana that doesn't make me high or sleepy? I don't want the kind with any THC. I want to feel less pain, but I need to be able to function."

A pure pain reliever without side effect would be a panacea, and a dream come true. In reality, CBD and THC are believed to have a synergistic effect, meaning that when they are used in conjunction, they are more effective together than they are alone.

Most patients do not obtain significant relief from CBD products alone. This means that they do need to take products with some THC content. To minimize side effects, I encourage patients to try products with lower ratio of THC first. If needed, patients can increase the THC ratio slowly, and titrate it up for a desirable effect to ease their pain.

It is a balancing act of pain relief and side effects. This process often takes some time and effort, requiring frequent return visits to the dispensary to try different products.

In addition to the potential lengthy trial and error process, the high cost of the medical marijuana products further adds another layer of frustration to patients. It is one thing to spend ten dollars on a drug that turns out to be ineffective. It is yet another if one spends a hundred dollars on a bottle of medical marijuana tincture, which turns out to do nothing for the pain.

Medical insurance in the U.S. doesn't cover any cost associated with medical marijuana. In fact, at this point, in time, all sales at dispensaries must be made in cash or debit card payment because of the federal regulation issues. Banks are regulated under the federal law. Since medical marijuana is federally illegal, banks are reluctant to handle any monetary transactions related to marijuana.

If the purchased medical marijuana product does not work, that hard-earned money would be gone. This financial stress has dampened the spirits of a good portion of my patients who can potentially obtain significant benefit, from using medical marijuana on a regular basis.

One of my patients spent over one thousand dollars on medical marijuana but still could not find a type that was truly effective, so she had to give it up. Another patient told me that medical marijuana was helpful, and he was able to stop taking oxycodone while using medical marijuana. However, he had to spend about three hundred dollars per month on the product, compared to ten dollars co-pay for his monthly oxycodone prescription. Simply because of financial reasons, he chose to go back to oxycodone instead.

For chronic pain patients, their disease and suffering have often reduced their productivity and salary earning ability. The guilt of not sharing their household responsibility or being a bread winner is already problematic. These patients are unwilling to become a bigger financial burden to their families, even if medical marijuana would be a superior choice over opioids or suffering.

AS MORE OF my patients became certified to use medical marijuana, I learned from each experience. Just like any other medication, it worked like a miracle for some of my patients; it did not help at all for others.

For most people, medical marijuana can offer some relief and benefit in many situations. Like every other drug, it has its side effects, such as dizziness, drowsiness, appetite changes, mood swings, and chronic lethargy. One should never drive or perform tasks requiring focus and mental acuity while using medical marijuana. Those who should not use it are people with heart disease, pregnant women and those who have a history of psychosis.

For those patients who choose to use medical marijuana on a regular basis, they encounter new and peculiar problems. After purchasing their product of choice, while still in the dispensary, consumption is not permitted. When walking out onto the federally funded sidewalk, consumption is not permitted.

So, patients have a state-protected right to purchase medical marijuana, but nowhere to actually consume it, but in the privacy of their homes.

In addition, when patients travel, I caution them not to bring their medical marijuana across the state line where it is not legalized. When patients travel via airplanes, which are under federal regulation, patients can potentially get into legal trouble if they carry their medical marijuana with them.

For those patients, I often have to give them a small prescription of opioids to cover their pain management during their vacations or trips. The bottom line is, one may have the state right to purchase and use marijuana, but take extra caution as to where to carry and consume it.

> "The art of medicine consists in amusing the patient while nature cures the disease." — Voltaire

A Day at the Weed Farm

DURING THE SUMMER of 2019, I was invited to visit PharmaCannis, a cannabis pharmaceutical manufacturing corporation in Montgomery, New York. PharmaCannis LLC, was one of five companies approved by the state to grow and sell medical marijuana at the time.

Along the sparsely populated roads in Montgomery, New York, sits a one-story low-slung beige building that gives no clue as to what is encompassed inside, but a large green cannabis leaf on the locked door to the main entrance allows you to make an assumption.

PharmaCannis is deliberately private about its product, as it is heavily regulated.

The product made at the pharmaceutical house is of a medical grade that is grown, cultivated, harvested, divided into strains, packaged, and sold to dispensaries throughout the state of New York.

Our group of seven visitors, mostly curious medical providers like myself, were directed to put on synthetic disposable gowns and booties, to protect the plants that are grown from seed to sale. Current Good Manufacturing Practices—CGMP—are strictly followed to comply with OSHA and State safety measures.

We were led to nurseries, all of enormous size. Each nursery has plants in different stages of growing cycles. Baby plants are cut from the mother plants which are labeled with the same bar code ID as the mother plants. This ID will follow each plant for its entire life cycle. Each batch of medical marijuana product can be traced back to the mother plant.

Cannabis plants take about eight to ten weeks to grow and mature. Sophisticated sensors and computer programs in the rooms constantly measure and control temperature, humidity, and lighting in the nursery to ensure the best conditions for the best crop yield possible.

Cannabis is a flowering plant. When grown for medicine, the flowers, also known as buds of the female plant, are cured, resulting in what we generally regard as cannabis, or "marijuana." Therefore, most plants in the farm are female. In fact, growers keep male plants away from female plants because when the females are fertilized, they will use up energy making seeds instead of making flowers.

As the plants develop, the flowers grow larger and more colorful, and they grow together in bunches. The flowers are made up of "sugar leaves," which are green buds covered in crystals.

As the plant progresses through the flowering stages, the buds get larger, and the flowers change colors. The buds and the resinous crystals are the trichomes. These make kief and are what smell the strongest.

One nursery room had row after row of maturing female cannabis plants, with crystals forming on the flowers and sugar leaves.

"Aaaah, it must be what heaven looked and smelled like," one of the visitors with us said. We all laughed and perhaps it was from taking a whiff of the cannabis "perfume." Although I started to get used to the pungent smell of marijuana, I still have not learned to like it. All of us were glad to get this firsthand experience and try to learn about these so-called "heavenly" plants.

Once mature, the plants are sent to a room nearby where the buds and crystal-bearing sugar leaves are trimmed, put on trays, and dried.

After viewing the drying room, we watched how the ethanol or carbon dioxide extractors processed the plants to create the final marijuana products that the consumer desires, including tinctures, sprays, oil for vape pens, and capsules. Different strains of cannabis plants produce different ratios of THC vs CBD in their final products.

According to Nathaniel S. Kendle, Manager of Operations at PharmaCannis, "The recent development of new technology has enabled researchers to study and understand the different organic compounds of cannabis called cannabinoids.

By individually isolating these cannabinoids from each plant, scientists have been able to investigate them further and study their effects on the body. Although over a hundred different cannabinoids have been identified so far, we are still in the beginning stages of understanding their full potential."

As these cannabinoids are studied and better understood, some of them are added back to the final marijuana products. For example, Turpenoids, the element that gives cannabis its distinctive scent, are pulled out in the activation process and added back at the end in a controlled fashion, to provide a more diversified taste, patient experience, and disease treatment efficacy. As technology improves, more forms of medical marijuana will be available on the market.

As I learned more about medical marijuana and have more patients using different types of it, I feel much more comfortable adding it as another tool to my repertoire to help my patients manage their pain.

Yet, some patients are offended when I suggest it to them for treatment. Some still worry that marijuana is a habit-forming substance that could result in chemical dependence.

More than 1.5 billion people in the world regularly suffer from chronic pain, and they're typically prescribed opioid pain relievers to manage their symptoms. But what happens when patients supplement their pain relievers with cannabis?

Researchers wanted to find out what effect both drugs had and whether they led to more addictive behaviors or harder drug use. They released their remarkable findings in the May 18, 2018, issue of Leafly.com. By examining data from 273 registered medical marijuana patients at a clinic in Michigan, the results showed that using medical marijuana did not increase the likelihood of abusing alcohol or other drugs.

One of the lead authors of the study, Brian Perron, an Associate Professor at the School of Social Work at the University of Michigan, noted the following:

"In those states where medical marijuana is legal, physicians should be aware that the drug is a potentially safer and more effective treatment than opioids."

In April 2018, Sanjay Gupta, MD., Associate Chief of the Neurosurgery Department, Assistant Professor of Neurosurgery at the Emory School of Medicine and Former Chief CNN medical Correspondent and 60 Minutes Reporter published an open letter to the United States Attorney General, Jeff Sessions.

In the letter, published on the CNN website, Dr. Gupta writes[19]:

> I feel obligated to share the results of my five-year-long investigation into the medical benefits of the cannabis plant. Not only can cannabis work for a variety of conditions such as epilepsy, multiple sclerosis and pain, sometimes, it is the only thing that works.
>
> Researchers from the Rand Corp., supported by the National Institute on Drug Abuse, conducted "the most detailed examination of medical marijuana and opioid deaths to date" and an approximately 20% decline in opioid overdose deaths between 1999 and 2010 in states with legalized medical marijuana and functioning dispensaries . . . Though it is too early to draw a cause-effect relationship, these data suggest that medicinal marijuana could save up to 10,000 lives every year.

19   https://hightimes.com/news/dr-sanjay-gupta-writes-letter-jeff-sessions-about-cannabis/

In short, Dr. Gupta concluded that medical marijuana has great potential to help people. He, like many people, had turned himself from a skeptic to an advocate, through learning about marijuana. I certainly hope he has ignited more interest in this topic and encouraged people to be more open minded regarding the use of medical marijuana. This is heady information to consume, and it makes it easier for me to explain to my patients who are willing to try medical marijuana.

Increasing number of states has legalized the use of medical marijuana for those who suffer chronic pain. The effort to legalize medical marijuana at the federal level is ongoing. With time, the medical community will accumulate more scientific and clinical data. This will help to educate everyone, including physicians, patients, pharmaceutical companies, and policy makers.

Just like Dr. Gupta, it took time and effort for me to learn about medical marijuana over the past few years. I converted myself from a reluctant bystander to an active advocator for the drug. I believe medical marijuana will gradually become more accessible, affordable, and convenient to use for those who find it helpful for their chronic pain and other medical issues.

In Arabic its name means "belt of fire," while in Spanish it means "small snake." In Hindi, it means "big rash" in Norwegian its name is helvetesild, literally "hell's fire."

The Virus that Lurks Within

"I DON'T EVEN remember having chicken pox," Gregg said when he showed me the rash that circled halfway around his torso.

I examined the angry blisters on his back and chest. "You obviously had chicken pox when you were little, and this is an unfortunate reoccurrence of the virus."

Gregg showed up at my office with a typical case of shingles on his torso. I am usually not the one who would first diagnose the condition. Patients often go to their primary care doctors or dermatologists because of the rash. But Gregg had been my long-term patient for his chronic low back pain. He was able to get an earlier appointment with me. He came to my office as soon as he could.

Shingles is also known as herpes zoster, a viral disease characterized by a full skin rash with blisters in a localized area. The earliest symptoms of shingles, which include headaches and a fever, are nonspecific, and may result in an incorrect early diagnosis. These symptoms are commonly followed by sensations of burning, itching, over sensitivity, or a tingling, pricking, or numbness in the affected areas. The disease can be mild to extreme and can be interspersed with quick stabs of agonizing pain.

Shingles is due to a reactivation of varicella-zoster virus, also known as chickenpox, within a person's body. The disease initially manifests itself as chickenpox, often during childhood. Once the disease has resolved, the virus may remain inactive in nerve cells, most commonly in spinal nerves. When it reactivates, it travels from the nerve cell body to the nerve endings in the skin, producing blisters. That is why shingles most commonly occurs on the torso. Each spinal nerve in the upper back runs its course from the spine to the chest. The blisters follow this pattern and produce a band-like area of pain and rash.

At first, the rash appears similar to the first appearance of hives. However, unlike hives, shingles cause skin changes normally resulting in a stripe or belt-like pattern that is limited to one side of the body and does not cross the mid-line.

The name shingles is a root word from Zoster which comes from Greek zōstēr, meaning "belt" or "girdle" after the characteristic belt-like dermatomal rash. The common name for the disease, shingles, derives from the Latin cingulus, a variant of Latin cingulum meaning "girdle."

If the virus is initially dormant then reactivates in other nerve cells, shingles may have additional symptoms and patterns, depending on the location involved. The trigeminal nerve is also a common target. Out of the three branches that the trigeminal nerve has, the branch that controls the eye is the most likely afflicted. When the virus is reactivated in this nerve branch, it is termed zoster ophthalmicus. The skin of the forehead, upper eyelid, and the orbit of the eye may be affected.

Zoster ophthalmicus occurs in approximately 10 to 25 percent of the cases. In few people, symptoms may cause chronic eye inflammation, actual loss of vision, and debilitating pain.

If the rash has appeared on the chest, identifying this disease requires only a visual examination, since very few diseases produce a rash in such specific pattern. When the rash is absent, shingles can be difficult to diagnose.

Risk factors for shingles virus reactivation include old age, poor immune function, and having had chickenpox before eighteen months of age. How the virus remains in the body or subsequently reactivates is not as yet well understood.

Weeks before the shingles onset, Gregg underwent surgery for coronary artery bypass grafts. Although he healed well from the intricate cardiac procedure, his immune system was threatened by the stress of his surgery. The varicella zoster virus that had been sleeping inside Gregg's body for years finally got its chance to wake up to produce the shingles.

"Why does it hurt so much? It's just a rash," Gregg asked. "I thought I could deal with pain well, because I am used to managing my chronic back problems. But this is like nothing else. It constantly burns, stabs, like electrical shocks. I can't sleep. I can't eat. I am so miserable. How can anyone live this way?"

I have seen my share of patients in my office for shingles-related pain. They stand out as a group of their own, because they are usually the most unhappy patients.

Roger, a ninety-three-year-old retired cardiologist, suffered from post-herpetic neuralgia, which is a chronic form of pain related to shingles. When I asked him to describe his pain, Roger said, "Pain from shingles is unusual. No matter how I describe it to you, you will never understand, Dr. Shue. The moment you experience it, if you ever do, you will immediately and completely understand what it is. It is so bad. It actually makes me think about suicide."

No, I was not surprised to hear what Roger said to me. In fact, my patients with chronic severe pain from shingles were the ones who most frequently told me, "I can't stand it anymore. I just want to die."

Roger is probably right. I may never understand what kind of pain shingles can cause, but I knew it was important to treat Gregg early and aggressively to avoid the development of post-herpetic neuralgia.

The aims of treatment in the acute phase, such as in Gregg's situation, are to limit the severity and duration of a shingles episode and reduce complications, including a secondary bacterial infection of the rash and skin lesions.

Anti-viral medication, such as acyclovir, can reduce the severity and duration of disease if it is started within seventy-two hours of the appearance of the rash. Corticosteroids, anticonvulsants, such as gabapentin, NSAIDS, and even opioids may be used to help with the acute pain.

It is estimated that about one-third of people, worldwide, develop shingles at some point. While more common among older people, children may also get the disease. Fortunately, shingles in children is often less painful. The condition has a strong relationship with increasing age, because cellular immunity declines as people grow older.

People not only are more likely to get shingles as they age, but also the disease tends to be more severe. About half of those living to age eighty-five will have at least one attack, and about five percent will have more than one attack.

The painful blisters eventually become cloudy or darkened, and crust over within seven to ten days. The pain usually subsides within three to five weeks, along with the healing of the rash.

However, about one in five people develop ongoing nerve damage, which can last for months or even years. Unfortunately, Gregg was one of this twenty percent.

Over the next three months, he returned a few times for follow-up. Although his rash completely healed, his pain continued. He had developed post-herpetic neuralgia.

To prevent and treat the symptoms of post-herpetic neuralgia, the American Academy of Neurology recommends a combination of treatment options, including: antidepressant drugs, specifically tricyclic antidepressants such as amitriptyline; anticonvulsants, such as gabapentin (Neurontin) or pregabalin (Lyrica); pain medications, either anti-inflammatory drugs like ibuprofen, or even opioids; topical anesthetics, such as lidocaine gels or patches, which should be applied to healed and intact skin only; capsaicin, which is the active ingredient in chili peppers, also has intriguing value.

The list seems to give patients and physicians a good variety of treatment choices. However, in reality, post-herpetic neuralgia, can be resistant to treatments and is particularly challenging to manage. Often, when we try patients on an antidepressant or anticonvulsant, we need to wait a few weeks to gauge if the medication is effective. If not, dosage needs to be increased and we must wait another week or so. If the patient is still not feeling better, we must switch to another type of medication and start the process all over again.

This can be very frustrating for both the patient and the doctor. The pain is often relentless, searing, and unbearable. Patients sometimes feel like they are guinea pigs, being put through experiment after experiment, shooting in the dark. They are unable to sleep due to pain and anxiety. They cannot work or even take care of themselves, because their pain overtakes their minds and energy. The process is often compounded by physical exhaustion, desperation, and depression.

Some patients, like Gregg, are unable to have meaningful relief from any oral or topical medications.

After weeks of unsuccessful treatment, I sat down with Gregg to review his options.

"Gregg, unfortunately, we have tried multiple medications and topicals for your shingles. Nothing has made you feel better. You have two choices. One is to give it more time and keep trying other medications at different dosages. The other is to consider an epidural steroid injection in the mid-back area. The goal of the procedure is to place cortisone close to the nerve root where the virus and the inflammation are located. Because pain is related to the inflammation of the nerve root, by the anti-inflammatory action of the cortisone, the nerve root may calm down and that may lessen your pain."

According to the article named "Herpes Zoster and Post-herpetic Neuralgia: Practical Consideration for Prevention and Treatment" by Young Hoon Jeon, published in 2015, interventional treatments, including epidural steroid injections, and other nerve blocks, have limited evidence to show they are effective treatments for post-herpetic neuralgia, in providing long-term relief[20].

On the other hand, guideline published in 2021 by the CMS (Center for Medicare and Medicaid Services) supported the utilization of epidural steroid injections for post herpetic neuralgia.

I want to make sure Gregg is fully informed, when comparing his treatment options.

"You may get better if we inject steroid in your mid-back by epidural injection. This treatment is controversial, but in my experience, about half of patients were able to get meaningful relief. There are risks involved in the procedure itself, which includes bleeding, infection, and even spinal cord injury."

20   https://pubmed.ncbi.nlm.nih.gov/26175877/

Gregg initially shook his head. "Too risky."

Then I explained the pros and cons to him. "Most doctors believe that doing the steroid injection sooner would give patients better results than waiting longer."

After some contemplating, Gregg grudgingly decided to take the chance. He was desperate. We proceeded with a thoracic steroid epidural injection at the level of T10, where his spinal nerve was irritated by the virus.

Two weeks later, Gregg returned and happily announced that his pain was reduced by half. He still had some discomfort but was able to sleep better.

"You don't understand how life is so good when I can sleep." he said with relief. "Pain is still there, but I am a happy man again."

I could not help but think to myself: What can pain do to people? When it hurts so much, life must be put on hold. How does pain put things in perspective for us? Happiness, sometimes, is just to have less pain to allow for a good night sleep. When we are so busy pursuing things that we think should make us happy, how much do we pay attention to the happiness that we take for granted but is a luxury for many others?

Gregg's pain further reduced after a second thoracic epidural steroid injection, a month later. His pain finally became manageable, and he was able to stop taking medication for it on a regular basis.

I was extremely happy with Gregg's progress, but I warned him to be vigilant because he could get shingles again. I also urged him to discuss with his primary care physician about shingles vaccination.

In fact, whenever I have the opportunity, I encourage my patients who are fifty years or older to talk to their doctors about getting vaccinated against shingles. I have seen enough suffering. Anything that can be done to prevent shingles should be considered.

In January 2018, the CDC officially recommended that adults fifty and over, including people who are unsure about their chicken pox history, get the new vaccine to prevent this painful, blistering disease.

There are currently two kinds of vaccines for shingles. In October 2017, the FDA approved the new shingles vaccine, Shingrix. Shingrix is more than 90 percent effective at preventing shingles and post-herpetic neuralgia in all age groups. Zostavax, the other kind of vaccine, lowers the odds of getting shingles by 51 percent, and of post-herpetic neuralgia by 67 percent. It's less effective in people ages seventy and older.

Gregg obtained the Shingrix vaccine and has been doing well ever since. Surely, he suffered terribly from the condition for the few months beforehand, but early treatment with medication and interventional pain management injections finally put his mind and body at ease.

Regrettably, this is not the case for Roger, my ninety-three-year-old-cardiologist patient, who developed shingles and continued to suffer long after the rash and active stage had passed.

Post-herpetic neuralgia is rare in people under fifty and the symptoms wear off in a reasonable amount of time. In older people, the pain wears off more slowly, but even in people over age seventy, 85 percent were pain-free a year after their shingles outbreak.

When Roger came to my office, he had already suffered from post-herpetic neuralgia for more than two years. Roger's blessed longevity, however, probably puts him at odds of the pain resolving on its own.

To make things more difficult, his shingles occurred in his scalp, behind his right ear. This location made any use of topical patches or cream difficult, especially since he had gracefully retained a good head of hair.

We went over Roger's treatment options. Since he had no success with medication but never tried any interventional treatments, we decided to try a steroid injection into the superficial nerves in the scalp. The steroid injection did not help. It was not surprising, because steroid injections are thought to be more efficacious if they are administered in the first six months. The effectiveness diminishes as the waiting period increases. This is believed to happen when the nerve inflammation becomes chronic and irreversible. Two years was probably too long for the steroid injection to be beneficial for Roger. He was not a candidate for epidural injections either due to the location of his afflicted nerve.

"Roger, I wish I had a silver bullet here, but I don't."

I sat down and discussed the situation with him again. "You are taking oxycodone every day for your pain. It would be fine if you did not have side effects. The constipation and dizziness from the opioids are making you miserable. The dizziness limits your activity level. If you had a fall, that would be really terrible. Would you be willing to give a change to something entirely new?"

"What is it? I am willing to try anything and everything," Roger said.

"Medical marijuana, Roger, I think you should try medical cannabis."

I explained to Roger that I have witnessed some significant success with medical marijuana use for other patients. Specifically, medical marijuana may offer him relief without the side effect of severe constipation that opioids gave him.

Roger was open-minded. He tried and found that medical marijuana offered him relaxation and pain relief. He was able to sleep better throughout the night, which he was unable to do for years. He was careful not to use it during the day, because he wanted to maintain his ability to drive. Yes, he still had his driver's license and was driving locally on a regular basis, at age ninety-three.

Pain relief for Roger was hardly perfect. When one has a severe persistent chronic pain caused by the virus that lurks within, we try to balance everything and make the best of it.

> "The most important thing in communication is hearing what isn't said." — Peter Drucker

Alvin's Struggle With Cancer

ALVIN WAS IN his late seventies and was referred to me by his oncologist. He had been taking a large amount of opioids at the behest of his cancer doctor.

"My doctor said that the amount of pain pills I am taking is beyond his specialty and I needed to see a pain management doctor to get my medication, so I chose you," Alvin explained.

"Who put you on this amount of medication?" I asked.

"My cancer doctor did. When I first went to see him for my cancer treatment, I was taking pain pills for my low back pain and my cancer pain, and he said it was not enough. He doubled my medication and I felt much better. Since then, I have been taking the same amount."

"How is your cancer treatment going and where is your pain?" I asked. Alvin's record showed that he had history of lung cancer that was currently stable.

"My lung cancer is quiet at the moment; I don't have any pain from it. I only have pain in my low back. My low back is the reason why I am taking my pain pills."

I explained to Alvin that opioids were important for treating cancer-related pain. However, it wasn't recommended for chronic use for non-cancer pain. I proceeded to give him a stern lecture regarding the importance of tapering down opioids, and be open-minded toward other treatment options if he wished to be a patient of mine.

"But why did my oncologist double my pills?"

"That was because you had ongoing pain from your lung cancer at the time. Now that your cancer is not bothering you, we need to minimize your pain medication use. This will prevent your body from getting used to the pain pills. Should you develop more pain problems later, the pills would work better."

Alvin was not happy about this situation, but grudgingly consented to my plan.

I presented him with a narcotic contract. If he came to me for pain management, he needed to strictly follow directions. He could not take more medication than he was prescribed.

Alvin was a stoic man; he came to me every month. I could tell that he did not like giving up his pain pills as I slowly but surely reduced his narcotic prescriptions. Sometimes, he would shake his head, but never with complaint or a demand for more medication.

Other than refilling his medication, Alvin tried and was able to obtain some pain relief from steroid injections to his low back in my office.

Almost one year went by, when Alvin came to my office again.

"I have been feeling some new pain in my groin area. I used to have some bladder problems that would give me that kind of pain and now I wonder what is going on."

Upon further questioning, it turned out that Alvin had not been keeping up with his regular follow up appointments with his oncologist. I instructed him to immediately go see his oncologist and urologist to make sure things were okay. This time, I kept his pain medication at the same level and did not reduce it.

I did, in fact, worry if Alvin's lung cancer was rearing its ugly head again. When I got the call from his oncologist's nurse practitioner, my heart sank. The newest C-T scan showed his cancer had metastasized to almost everywhere in his body.

"We think that Alvin has about three months to live," his oncologist said when he got on the phone.

"He is in terrible shape and severe pain, and we suggested that he enter a hospice for palliative care, but he would rather be treated by you. We just wanted you to know the latest update on him. He said you would care."

I felt my stomach churning after I hung up with the doctor. Why did Alvin remain quiet about his escalating pain? Why did he suffer in silence?

I immediately called Alvin to discuss his management plan. "Alvin, why didn't you say something if your pain has been getting so much worse?"

"I respect you as a specialist in pain management," he replied. "I signed the contract in order to follow your directions. I have to tell you that you are the best pain management doctor I have ever encountered, and I have been to quite a few. But if I asked you for more medication, I was afraid that you would not keep me as a patient anymore because I broke the contract."

A wave of complex emotions came upon me. He chose to grin and bear it, because he wanted to follow every word on the narcotic contract. On the other hand, I hadn't lived up to his trust to reduce his suffering. I blamed myself for not making sure that he understood the real purpose of the contract, I also wish I was able to pick up signs of his decline sooner. "Alvin, the contract said that you should tell me what is really going on with you. If we don't have a completely truthful conversation, I cannot do my part to treat and ease your pain. From now on, I need you to tell me exactly how you are doing and how you feel."

Virtually all patients with cancer have recurrent episodes of acute pain, which may result from surgery, invasive procedures, or complications, such as a bone fracture due to cancer invasion.

In addition, chronic pain that is severe enough to warrant opioid therapy is experienced by 30 to 50 percent of patients undergoing active anti-cancer therapy and by 75 to 90 percent of those with advanced disease.

The bottom line is that causes of chronic pain are complicated. How likely a patient would have pain and how much pain would be experienced vary with the type of cancer, stage and extent of disease, prior treatments, and other factors.

I explained to Alvin that since his cancer was the main cause of his pain, the treatment and management would be much different. Our primary goal for him would be to maintain his quality of life as much as possible.

To treat Alvin's pain adequately was not only a medical issue and my personal concern. In fact, a physician has an ethical and a legal duty to relieve patients' suffering.

The evidence that physicians and nurses do not treat pain adequately began to appear in the medical literature over thirty years ago.

Multitudes of factors can lead to inadequate pain treatments. There is a lack of accountability for providing effective pain relief. Healthcare providers worry about regulatory scrutiny of their prescribing practices, given the ongoing opioid crisis. Doctors are also concerned about the risks of addiction, tolerance, and adverse side effects associated with opioids.

The outcome of two legal cases—the *James* case and the *Bergman* case—had shown the medical community that its duty to relieve suffering is not only an ethical one but is enshrined in law.

In 1991, a North Carolina jury awarded fifteen million dollars in compensatory and punitive damages to the family of Henry James. Mr. James was a nursing home patient. A nurse refused to give him the opioids to relieve his pain, because of fear of the patient becoming addicted to the medication. The patient died a painful death from terminal metastatic prostate cancer. The jury found this action constituted a gross departure from acceptable care.[21]

In 1998, William Bergman was admitted to Eden Medical Center in Castro Valley, California, in severe pain, under the care of Dr. Chin. A chest X-ray, combined with a long history of smoking, was strongly suggestive of lung cancer. Mr. Bergman declined further treatment, went home, and received hospice care. He died within a week of discharge. Mr. Bergman's family did not think that appropriate pain management was provided to Mr. Bergman for his severe pain and suffering during his hospitalization. Mr. Bergman's family filed suit against Dr Chin and Eden Medical Center. Eden

21   https://open.mitchellhamline.edu/cgi/viewcontent.
cgi?referer=&httpsredir=1&article=1839&context=wmlr

Medical Center settled before trial. On June 13, 2001, the jury returned a verdict against Dr Chin of $1.5 million.[22]

These verdicts have shown us that there is a standard of care for pain management, a significant departure from which constitutes not only malpractice but gross negligence.

What is under treating pain, and what is over treating pain? With the pendulum of opioid prescribing swinging back and forward over the past few decades, both experts and the general public may have drastically different standard of care in mind. Above all, it is unequivocal that a doctor's duty is to relieve suffering, especially for cancer pain patients. Such was the case when I attempted to meet the critical needs of Alvin with his metastasized cancer. His total trust in me made me feel the heaviness on my shoulders.

I gradually increased Alvin's opioids. When he was taking four times as his original dosage, the pain lessened, but he suffered the unpleasant side effects.

"I feel like a zombie when I take them," Alvin said. "I don't want to live the rest of my life like this. I want to feel like a human being."

When cancer spreads to many organs, as Alvin's had, patients usually have multiple pain sources, creating different types of distress. Patients often require large amount of opioids.

In many countries, since 1977, oral morphine has been used in Hospices and Palliative Care Units as the drug of choice for the management of chronic cancer pain. Morphine provides effective pain relief. It is simple to be administered and is cheap. Moreover, morphine is the only opioid analgesic considered in the World Health Organization essential drug list for adults and children with pain. Other opioids, including oxycodone, the fentanyl patch, methadone, oxymorphone, just to name a few, are widely used for cancer pain treatment.

With chronic and high dosage of opioid use, many patients develop significant side effects such as constipation, nausea, vomiting, urinary retention, itching, drowsiness, confusion, and hallucinations. In some cases, when side effects from opioids become unacceptable, doctors may have to reduce opioid dose to alleviate side effects. This is when alternative approaches, such as a nerve block, can be valuable.

For example, patients with pancreatic cancer, usually suffer from severe and unrelenting abdominal and back pain. A constellation of nerve fibers called the celiac plexus is responsible to convey pain from the abdomen to the brain. By injecting the area around the celiac plexus with local anesthetic, or sometimes other medicines, such as anti-inflammatory steroids, it may be possible to reduce this pain for some period of time.

22   https://www.sfgate.com/health/article/Doctor-found-reckless-for-not-relieving-pain-2909969.php#

This procedure is often done under Xray guidance by interventional pain management physicians like me, or under endoscopic ultrasound guidance by gastroenterologists. To obtain longer termed relief, phenol and alcohol can be used in the chemical destruction of the nerve fibers.

Although chemical neurolysis of the celiac plexus can be an effective means to treat pancreatic cancer pain, it is a risky procedure. The targeted nerves are seated next to major blood vessels and vital structures, where heavy bleeding and bowel incontinence are often possible side effects. As a result, these treatments are only offered to terminally ill patients as a last resort to make their final days more comfortable.

For Alvin, he did not have the option for such nerve blocks, even if he would like to take the risk of side effects. His pain was in his chest wall, ribs, abdomen, groin, and spine. There was not a single bundle of nerves that we could work on to numb or reduce his pain.

For about one to two percent of patients, their cancer pain can be persistent and severe, despite all conventional strategies and medications. For these patients, spinal analgesia administered via an intrathecal pump can be helpful.

Intrathecal drug delivery, or "pain pump," is a method of giving medication directly to the spinal cord. A small pump with a medication reservoir is surgically placed under the skin of patient's belly. The pump is programmed to automatically deliver medication through a catheter to the area around the spinal cord. Because the spinal cord is much more sensitive to the action of pain medications, pain can be controlled with a much smaller dose than is needed taking the same medication orally.

For example, if a patient is using 100mg morphine pills each day, he or she would only need about 1-5mg morphine given in the intrathecal pump.

The goal of a drug pump is to better control pain and reduce oral medications; thus drastically reducing their associated side effects.

The pump can be programmed to release different amounts of medication at different times of the day, depending on patient's needs. It stores the information about medication prescription in its memory. Doctors can easily review this information and adjust if needed. When the reservoir is empty, the doctor or nurse refills the pump via a special port on top of the reservoir.

I discussed the option of an Intrathecal Morphine Pump with Alvin. The pump could probably eliminate his need to take pills all day long and allow him to live a more functional life.

Alvin was excited about the intrathecal morphine pump. I referred him to a local neurosurgeon who routinely performs this surgery. Morphine pump implants and managements are usually done in academic centers because doctors in private practices rarely have the resources and support to manage these patients' requirements.

Alvin went ahead and made arrangements with the neurosurgeon, but pre-operative tests indicated that his cancer had progressed to affect his breathing and heart function. The neurosurgeon determined that it would be unsafe for him to undergo any kind of surgery, including the morphine pump for pain control.

The next time I saw Alvin, he was wheelchair bound. During our time together, I convinced him to use medical marijuana which might have been helpful, and he did although he still required a large amount of opioids which continued to give him side effects.

"Pain management and palliative care are two different fields," I tried to explain to Alvin. "I cannot tell you how honored I feel to have your trust, and I treat you like family. Now I really think you should have hospice involved in your care, as well. I already called them and made sure that even if you start care with them, that you can call me anytime. I will still be your doctor."

Alvin finally agreed to get hospice care at home.

"But I would still come to see you," he said as his face lit up with a smile. It made me feel so much better that his face was peaceful, and calm.

That was the last time I saw Alvin. His cancer had destroyed his bones and gave him a hip fracture, just from walking. He was unable to have surgery and required a large dosage of intravenous morphine for the severe pain.

Soon after that, Alvin died peacefully in hospice care, and I mourned.

I have lost a few patients over the years, from old age, disease, or accidents. No matter how many years I have been a physician; no matter how many deaths I have witnessed, I do not think I will ever get used to losing a patient, especially a patient with whom I have built a strong bond like the one I had with Alvin.

Looking back at my experience with him, one cannot emphasize more than I, that communication between doctor and patient is critical. Never be afraid to tell your doctor all that is bothering you. Chances are your doctor will be empathic and help to ease the problem to the best of their ability.

"You know, there's nothing damnable about being a strong woman." — Ginger Rogers

Bertha's Osteoarthritis

BERTHA WAS EIGHTY-FOUR years old when she showed up at my office for her scheduled appointment.

"Everything is hurting me, my shoulders, elbows, knees, hips. I don't know what's going on. My doctors never explained anything to me. What is wrong with me?"

Before I had a chance to answer, Bertha continued. "I was always so healthy. I was on the track team in high school and college. I was the captain of the softball team. I worked out every day. I walked and ran for miles every week. I never got married so I have always done everything for myself. I could handle everything in the house like a man. I shoveled snow on my own driveway. I mowed my lawn. I bought and handled all the furniture in the house myself. I had aches and pains over the years, but I am tough; I don't complain. Believe me. I am not a complainer. I have high tolerance for pain. I never had to take any pain medication. But these last couple of years, things just started to go downhill for me. Now I can't even move without my walker. I went to so many doctors. They all said that there was nothing they can do for me.

"I need new knees, new hips, new shoulders, new everything. But nobody is willing to do anything for me. They said I won't make it through any surgery alive."

While listening to Bertha, I sifted through her chart. My head was already spinning with her fiery and prolong monologue. On her chart, it said that she had suffered two heart attacks, a stroke, severe COPD, which usually means bad breathing problems from years of smoking.

Wow! I was bewildered and thought to myself, Her lungs and breathing problems obviously are not that bad. Her stroke seems to have left all her speech processing centers intact. With all that she has gone through, she has miraculously preserved all her ability to chatter away without having to catch her breath or stop to think at all.

With her multiple and severe medical problems, it would be too risky to put her through elective surgeries, because of the possible complications from anesthesia, surgical trauma, and lengthy recovery. Bertha was in chronic severe pain, but she did not need new joints to survive. It would not make sense for her to risk her life to improve her pain. That would mean that surgeries that could give Bertha new knees and hips were out of the question for her.

Bertha clearly showed no signs of slowing down, and she continued. "I know exercises are important. I really cannot walk much anymore. But now it is summer. The weather is beautiful. I live not too far from the beach. I try to go swimming. You know, I need to leave my things on the beach. It is usually crowded on the beach. If I leave my things too far away from the water, it is hard for me to walk to them. I cannot really use my walker on the beach . . ."

After five minutes of detailing her swimming routine, she proceeded to tell me about her sick brother.

"You know, my sister-in-law died, and my brother is ninety years old, and he has dementia. He never had children, so I have to take care of him. I am too old to drive. That means I have to take the bus to see him every day. It is hard not to have good legs anymore. That's why I really to need to be able to move around better. I can't live like this. Why do I have pain everywhere? Nobody ever explained to me what's wrong with me."

Bertha provided me with X-rays and MRI reports of almost all the major joints in her body, ordered by different doctors, done at different times over the past five years. They all invariably showed moderate to severe osteoarthritis. By now, I was not surprised why she kept complaining and why nobody had explained things to her.

I stole a look at the clock. A forty-five-minute new patient consultation visit was already half-way gone before I had much chance to do my job. Bertha, I could imagine, also competed with other doctors for their time to talk.

"Bertha, what you have is osteoarthritis. It is all over your body in almost all of your joints."

I often see patients whose reports, conditions, and treatment options had not been explained well by other doctors when they were seen at my office. I always try to take time to give patients details about their medical conditions, pros, and cons of different treatment options. When I saw Bertha's eyes full of curiosity and ready to hear me out, I was ready to explain.

And I told her all she wanted to know. "Osteoarthritis, also known as wear-and-tear arthritis, happens when the natural cushioning cartilage between joints wears away. The bones of the joints rub against one another. The rubbing results in swelling, stiffness, decreases the ability to move and sometimes that motion forms bone spurs. While it can start in people's twenties, the chance of developing osteoarthritis increases after age forty-five."

"But I was fine at forty-five," she interrupted.

"Yes, and I'll explain why," I said calmly. "Almost everyone will eventually develop some degree of osteoarthritis. However, several factors increase the risk. The most common risk for osteoarthritis is age. And this is why: The ability of cartilage to heal decreases as a person gets older. Weight increases pressure on all the joints, especially the knees. Every pound of weight you gain, adds three to four pounds of extra weight on your knees."

At this point, Bertha had begun to really listen.

"Arthritis tends to run in families. Heredity might make a person more likely to develop osteoarthritis. Repetitive stress injuries are commonly seen in arthritis. People with certain occupations that include a lot of activity that can stress the joint, such as kneeling, squatting, or lifting heavy weights are more likely to develop osteoarthritis because of the constant pressure on the joint."

"That must be part of my problem," Bertha interjected.

"Athletes like you, who involved in strenuous training regimen long term are also at higher risk for developing osteoarthritis. However, regular moderate exercise strengthens joints and can decrease the risk of osteoarthritis. In fact, weak muscles around the knee can lead to osteoarthritis. Like everything else in life, moderation is the key while exercising.

"People with rheumatoid arthritis, on the other hand, the second most common type of the disease, are also more likely to develop osteoarthritis. People with certain metabolic disorders, such as iron overload or excess growth hormone, also run a higher risk of osteoarthritis. And gender is key. Women ages fifty-five and older are much more likely than men to develop osteoarthritis of the knee."

"But what can I do to make it better, Dr. Shue?"

"At this time, nobody can stop or reverse arthritis. However, we can manage symptoms with medications, lifestyle changes, physical and other therapies, and surgery. "I always recommend acetaminophen as first line medication treatment. One can take up to 1000mgs, three times a day safely, unless there is pre-existing liver disease. This means you can take two extra strength Tylenol, three times a day.

"NSAIDs, including ibuprofen up to 800mg three times a day, as well as naproxen up to 500mg twice a day, can be taken with food, as needed. You can also try stronger prescription NSAIDs, such as meloxicam, celecoxib, and diclofenac. NSAIDs work to reduce inflammation. Yet NSAIDs can cause stomach upset, cardiovascular problems, bleeding problems, and kidney damage. Therefore, use NSAIDs with caution. Avoid using them every day or long term. Topical NSAIDs, on the other hand, have fewer side effects and may relieve pain just as well.

"Regular gentle exercise that you do on your own, such as swimming or walking, is very important to strengthen the muscles around your joints, increase your range of motion and reduce the pain. You can follow exercises on the internet and do them at home. Start with five minutes a day and work to thirty minutes a day. If you need professional guidance, a physical therapist can work with you to create an individualized exercise program. An occupational therapist can also help you discover ways to do everyday tasks or do your job without putting extra stress on your already painful joints. For instance, a toothbrush with a large grip could make brushing your teeth easier if you have osteoarthritis in your fingers. A bench in your shower could help relieve the pain of standing if you have knee osteoarthritis. Tai Chi and yoga involve gentle exercises and stretches, combined with deep breathing."

"Tai Chi, huh? That's something I've never done."

"Many people use these therapies to reduce stress in their lives," I told her, "and research suggests that Tai Chi and yoga may reduce osteoarthritis pain and improve movement.

"If conservative treatments don't help, you may want to consider procedures, such as injections of corticosteroid in your joints to relieve pain. Injections of hyaluronic acid may also offer pain relief and better joint movements by providing some cushioning in your knees. Hyaluronic acid is similar to a component normally found in your joint fluid. It is like putting DW40 in a squeaky door hinge to make the door move more smoothly."

"Oh, boy. I definitely can use some DW40 in all of my joints!" Bertha laughed.

"If you didn't have a number of other medical issues, Bertha, when osteoarthritic pain is severe and persistent despite medications and injections, then it would be time to consider surgery for possible replacement joint procedures."

"Are you sure I can't have any surgery?"

"Surgery is out of the question, Bertha. We'll use hot and cold compresses, topical creams and ointment and acetaminophen, as needed. Please do the exercises at home since you did not want to spend the time or extra money in physical therapy, and we will consider steroid joint injections in your knees, hips, or shoulders, but only if you have severe flare ups of pain."

Bertha was satisfied when she left. She held my hands. "You were very thorough," she said happily. "You explained things so well. Nobody has done that for me. Thank you so much. I will surely be calling you when I need any treatment."

After about one hour of fighting for my chance to talk, I managed to say all I wanted to say and explain all I needed to explain to Bertha.

Two months later, Bertha came for a right hip steroid injection.

While I was getting my procedure tray and medication set up in the procedure room, Bertha started. "My right hip and groin are hurting me so much. I cannot walk or stand any longer. Nothing is working. Why do I have this pain? Dr. Shue, can you tell me why? Nobody has ever explained this to me."

I felt a dizziness in my head. Boy, did I still remember that one-hour long consultation. How could she seem to not remember it at all?

"Bertha, it is your osteoarthritis," I reminded her, then gathered my patience and gave her a quick explanation of the problem once more.

"You know, I try to keep myself active, Dr. Shue. The weather is nice. I live close to the beach. I would go swimming on the beach. But I have to leave my things on the beach . . ."

She went over her swimming routine and her sick brother yet again for the next twenty minutes or so, as I placed the needle under X-ray guidance in her right hip joint and gave her a steroid injection to calm down her hip pain. I put the bandage on and told her not to overuse her hips too much that day because the joint would be numb for a few hours due to the Lidocaine given together with the steroid. She would not feel pain in the joints but may damage them further if she would start running too many errands because she did not feel any pain in the hip due to the numbing medications . . .

All done! I was just about to quietly sneak out of the procedure room.

"Wait, Dr. Shue, wait a minute. Can I talk to you for a few minutes? I have a list of questions that I had written down on a piece of paper." Bertha fished out a wrinkled paper from her bag, full of her hand writings.

Oh, no! Now I really was feeling dizzy.

Over a short period of time, Bertha became quite the celebrity among my employees. Every one of my staff's eyes would go wide at the mention of her name. When her caller ID showed up on the phone, the staff member would have to take a deep breath before picking up the call. We all knew every medical problem she had, her swimming routine, her brother's health status, her complaint of no doctors ever explaining anything to her, her eternal questioning of what was wrong with her, because she would repeat everything, every time, regardless, if she was on the phone or in the office.

When I saw Bertha's name on my schedule, I would be overcome with a heavy sense of dread and foreboding. I had to mentally prepare myself. I would have a quick drink of water, do my yoga stretches, and take a deep breath, before I entered the "battleground."

Hypothetically speaking, to master the art of doctoring, I ought to be the leader during conversations with my patients. I should possess the ability to redirect them when they go on talking about things unrelated to their medical issues.

Somehow, my "divine" doctoring powers never worked with Bertha. My bag of tricks was useless with her. I did not want to complain, because I would be protesting against my own incompetence and inadequacy. I just wanted to hide.

Bertha was in my office again! Twenty minutes elapsed. Our conversation became dominated by Bertha's monologue, as usual. I tried to figure out my exit strategy. I was already forty-five minutes behind my schedule that afternoon. I could hardly focus as Bertha was jabbering away. Instead, I worried about the annoyed patients in the waiting room, my stack of charts that I had to complete, and the long list of phone calls that I had to make before going home.

So much work to do. Instead of doing real work, I was drowning in Bertha's ocean of chatter.

I stood up while nodding and smiling at Bertha. She kept talking. I opened the door and stepped one foot out. Bertha was still talking. By now, both of us were probably used to this routine, because this was what I had to do every time Bertha came to my office.

"Bertha, it was good seeing you today. We will chat some more next time."

Finally, I managed to quickly make my closing statement before she had the chance to blur out the next wave of words. I escaped and ran in to my office.

Just as I breathed a sigh of relief, to my shock, Bertha had followed me into my office.

It was unprecedented. I panicked.

Before I could think of how to get rid of her, she grabbed my hands and said, "I know you are busy. I just need a few more minutes. I wanted to thank you and your staff. Nobody ever wants to listen to me. You are the only ones to whom I can talk. I never got married. I don't have my own family. Now my brother has dementia so bad, he can't talk to me anymore.

"I have nobody to talk to. I sometimes come here just because I wanted to talk to you. I just want to thank you again."

I looked at Bertha, speechless. Something deep inside me was touched. I felt my face burning with guilt. I hugged Bertha, gently turned her around, and told her to be on her way.

Quality patient interaction and communication are essential to healthcare. However, physicians are under increasing pressure of efficiency and productivity. We have less time allocated for our patients. We also still need to keep the office running on time, which is the only fair way to treat other patients. To maintain a balance remains a constant challenge to physicians.

Platelet Rich Plasma Treatment
Or PRP
As It's Known in the Field

ALLISON, A PETITE slender woman in her late forties came into my office one sunny afternoon. As we began our consultation, she told me she worked as a correctional officer at a county facility. One day, as she was trying to break up a fight between two inmates, she was pushed and shoved, and her right knee slammed to the floor. From then on, she had experienced persistent and intense knee pain. To her surprise, her knee X-ray and MRI both showed moderate osteoarthritis.

"I have never had any knee problems before my fall," she said with concern. "I'm not overweight. I exercise regularly. I was shocked that my knee would look like that of an older person. For the past year, I diligently went to my physical therapy sessions and did my daily home exercises. I tried taking ibuprofen, naproxen, and prescription NSAIDS, but my knee still hurts—especially as soon as I stopped taking these medications. I then tried steroid injections and gel injections into the knee joint. I did feel better but only for a few weeks. I'm only in my forties, and I cannot possibly be taking pills every day and getting steroid injections every few months.

"I went to see a few orthopedists. They all told me that I probably would need a knee joint placement down the road. However, they told me that I am too young to have it done now. I need to wait at least five to ten years, or until I retire. But, what about now? I still need to live my life."

I asked her more about her job. She told me, as a correctional officer, she's on her feet all day long, carrying a belt with her equipment and protective gear that would weigh no less than fifteen pounds.

Wear and tear on the knees from the heavy belt; remaining on her feet long hours every day; working at her job since her twenties had finally caught up with Alison.

Allison tried all appropriate conservative therapies, including medications, physical therapy, both steroid and hyaluronic acid knee injections. She was deemed not to be candidate for a knee replacement surgery.

So, why did surgeons tell Alison she was too young to have surgery?

Joint replacements generally are very effective, allowing most people to return to active lives free of chronic pain. However, artificial joints cannot last forever. This means that the chance of needing a redo of the joint replacement is high if the first one is done at a young age.

Revision surgery is a longer and more complex procedure, it requires specialized tools and implants, as well as a surgeon with advanced technical skills. Doctors generally try to avoid revision surgeries for joint replacements.

There are two kinds of situations that would result in the need for repeated joint replacement surgery. One situation is when patients have infection develops in the joint after surgery. This is a thankfully rare occurrence. The other situation is more common. With long term use of an artificial joint, the bond between the bone and the implant loosens over time, or a component of the implant wears down. When this type of problem occurs, a revision surgery is needed to replace the original implant.

Based on many large studies of different joint implants, it is generally thought that around at least 90 percent of modern total knee replacements still function well fifteen to twenty years later. That number might be even higher for total hip replacements.

For relatively young patients like Allison, leading an active, productive lifestyle, chances are, they would need a second joint replacement surgery in the future if they were to undergo their first surgery before they turn fifty, because they are likely to live beyond the age of seventy years old. This is why Allison's orthopedist doctors were reluctant to offer her surgery at this point.

"Dr. Shue," Allison said plaintively, "that's why I came to see you. I am in this peculiar situation where medications and steroid injections are not helping enough, but I am not ready to have surgery. I have come so far to build a life for myself. I have a good career and a good family. I can't let my knee pain affect my work or my life."

During our conversion, I learned a few things about Alison's upbringing and childhood in the Bronx. She was the oldest of ten children in the family. Each of the ten children had a different father.

"We grew up like weeds, on our own," Alison said. "It still amazes myself how I managed to get a college degree and have such a nice job. My mom never even mentioned the word 'college' to me, ever. She couldn't care less. From a young age, I knew that I didn't want to follow my mother's footsteps. This desire was enough to push me to study and work hard. My friends would call me names and ridicule me. I didn't care. Now I am the one who has the final laugh. Some of my old friends are already gone. I mean gone." She looked at me to make sure I understood what she really meant.

I could only imagine what terrible things could happen to people when growing up with the wrong crowd.

It was impressive for Allison to have a college education, a stable marriage, and an aspiring career, growing up with hardly any parental support or a female role model. She quickly earned my respect and admiration.

"I would like to know if you can do PRP injections for my knee. I heard a lot of good things about it," Allison posed.

I was intrigued that she had specifically asked about platelet-rich plasma—also known as PRP.

Data has shown that there had been a significant rise in the use of PRP procedures for pain related to osteoarthritis of the hip and knee since 2009. I have certainly been seeing this trend in my own office. Patients like Allison, who was determined to avoid surgery for the time being, are most motivated to search for potential non-operative treatments. Patients who are concerned about risks and lengthy recovery course associated with surgeries are also interested in PRP injections.

In recent years, doctors have learned that the body has the potential to heal and regenerate. Platelet-rich plasma is thought to contain concentrated natural growth factors that human body uses to heal injured tissues.

What is plasma and what are platelets?

Plasma is the liquid portion of whole blood. It consists of mainly water and proteins. Platelets, also called thrombocytes, are blood cells that help stop bleeding when we have tissue injuries. Scientists and doctors think that platelet activation plays a key role in tissue healing in a human body.

What is platelet-rich plasma (PRP) and what are PRP injections?

Platelet-rich plasma (PRP) therapy uses **injections** of a concentration of a patient's own platelets to promote the healing of injured tendons, ligaments, muscles, and joints. PRP injections are prepared by collecting about fifty milliliters of a patient's own blood and processing it through a centrifuge to concentrate the platelets. The resulted product is then injected into the injured joints or tissue. Doctors believe that this process releases growth factors that increase the number of reparative cells in the injured area, which are essential to tissue repair. Ultrasound and X-Ray imaging are often used to guide the injections.

Platelet-rich plasma has been found in some studies to significantly enhance the healing process for shoulder pain caused by **rotator cuff tears,** for Achilles tendon ruptures, and for other acute soft-tissue injuries. PRP can also benefit people who have chronic tendonitis conditions, such as **tennis elbow or golfer's elbow.**

Some doctors believe that the key advantage of PRP injections is that they can improve functionality, while reducing the need for medication intake, such as NSAIDs and **opioids.** In addition, the side effects of PRP injections are minimal. Since the injections are created from a patient's own blood, this patient's body will unlikely reject or react negatively to them.

With medical advancements for the use of PRP therapy, doctors have expanded the kinds of medical conditions they can implement PRP to treat.

Evidence showing PRP therapy's benefit for mild to moderate osteoarthritis has been growing too.

With increasing popularity and sometimes favorable clinical data, more patients would come into my office, asking to try PRP injection. However, unfortunately, PRP injections are generally not covered by Medicare, Medicaid, or most commercial insurances, because insurance companies consider them to be "experimental."

The cost of a single PRP injection treatment ranges from a few hundred dollars to more than a thousand dollars, depending on which area is being treated and what special equipment doctor offices use.

While there is no consensus on how often PRP injections should be done, it is generally recommended to have a series of two to three injections, three to six months apart. The cost of PRP injections can quickly add up to thousands of dollars.

I became interested in PRP injections and regenerative medicine in the mid-2010s. However, because of lack of insurance coverage and the high cost of the procedure, I was unsure as to how to advise my patients with this experimental treatment. I always laid out the facts:

While there is minimal harm to inject something of your own blood back into your body, you have to understand that it may not work well because scientific data is not quite as strong as what I would like to see. You would have to be ready to spend this amount of money and make peace with yourself if you get no results.

Many patients would give up the idea of trying PRP due to the expense. Fortunately, Allison was in luck. Her knee pain was from wear and tear while working at the correctional facility. It was also made worse by the fall while working. Her knee pain treatment was covered under New York State Workman's Compensation Program. Allison's Workman's Compensation Insurance gave us the permission to perform a PRP injection for her right knee.

Shortly after her first visit, Allison came for her PRP injection appointment. I told her to drink lots of fluids in the morning and be well hydrated, because the first step of the procedure was to collect 50 milliliters of blood from her arm. The collection was the same to giving blood for a blood test.

The next step was for Allison to rest while the blood was processed by a centrifuge. A centrifuge is a device that spins at high speeds, which separates the solid from the liquid in whole blood. Heavier red blood cells settle in the bottom of the tube, while lighter weight plasma stays in the upper part of the tube. The layer with the most platelets is the three to seven millimeters of substance in the middle of the top and bottom layers. Regular blood contains about two hundred thousand platelets per milliliter, while platelet-rich plasma contains as much as five times that amount.

With the guidance of an X-Ray machine, the collected five milliliter PRP was immediately injected into Allison's right knee. This injection process and technique would be the same as a corticosteroid knee injection.

PRP can initially cause acute inflammation in the injection site. That acute inflammation can make patients feel sore and stiff for two to three days after injections. It takes time for the recruited reparative cells to move into the injured area and start the healing process.

Pain relief usually starts to occur within three to four weeks after the injection. Patients can continue to improve over a period of three to six months following a PRP injection.

To my delight, Allison reported improvement of her knee pain and her ability to tolerate working full time work when she returned to my office for a follow up visit in three months and then in six months. We repeated PRP injections on Allison every six to eight months. So far, she has been managing her reduced knee symptoms and was able to delay the need for a knee replacement surgery. I was happy to see this hard working and self-motivated woman able to keep on achieving her goals and enjoying her life.

With the success of Allison's case, I started talking to more patients regarding PRP injections, especially those who have potential insurance coverage. This is a safe treatment modality that could offer great potential for many patients.

There is growing evidence that supports PRP and regenerative medicine treatment in pain management, such as osteoarthritis of the hip and knee, tendinitis, neuropathic pain due to nerve injury or nerve disorder.

There is still a wide gap, nonetheless, between the promise and the reality of regenerative medicine in clinical practice that can only be bridged through basic scientific research. Clinical efficacy, patient safety, and cost-effectiveness are among the main considerations during further development of RPR and other regenerative medicine as an effective therapy for patients with a wide range of acute or chronic pain conditions.

> "The secret of change is to focus all of your energy.
> Not on fighting the old, but on building the new." — Socrates

IT'S TENNIS OR DIE!

OVER THE YEARS, I have seen different patients' reactions to the result of epidural injections. One told me, "The injection didn't work at all. My pain was only gone for six months. I don't want them anymore."

Another said, "I only feel better for one week after each treatment. I know you don't think I should have any more injections, but that one week is like holiday for me. I would feel like a completely different person. To me, it is worth the risk and the trouble to come for the treatment."

To treat, or not to treat? This is indeed a personal choice. A doctor's job is to help our patients make the best decision, given the circumstances.

Carol was an upbeat, active woman in her late seventies. She came to my office with the typical symptoms of nerve impingement from spinal stenosis, which is a degenerative spine disease. With aging and years of changes related to osteoarthritis and spine degeneration, the openings for the spinal nerves to exit out of the spinal column become smaller and smaller. This change is gradual and insidious. Eventually, the critical moment happens when the nerve is tightly surrounded by arthritic changes and bone spurs. When this becomes the case, any little irritation, such as a wrong turn, or picking up a gallon of milk aggravates the spinal nerve. All of a sudden, people may feel severe pain, seemingly out of nowhere.

That was exactly what happened to Carol, who became unhappy about the pain in her low back, shooting down both legs, which came out of nowhere. She chose to try lumbar epidural injections, anxious in getting rid of her symptoms so that she could go back to competitive tennis matches at her club.

Carol came for a follow-up appointment after she had a series of three epidural injections. While there is no scientific data consistently indicating what would be an optimal number of epidural injections, doctors generally would do a series of two or three over a year's time, which is accepted as the number that would provide good results for most patients. I always start with one, then bring the patient back to the office to see how much progress and pain relief are achieved. The patient and I go over options again to decide if more treatments should be performed.

"The pain in the back and leg is much better, but how come it still hurts? How come nothing is working for me?" Carol didn't try to hide her discontent. "I never had pain like this in more than seventy years of my life. I am not asking for much. All I am asking is for you to take this pain away so I can enjoy my tennis game with my friends."

"Carol, I understand that it is frustrating to deal with chronic pain. Even a single day feels too long having it. However, look how much progress you have already made." I tried to calm her down. "Spinal stenosis is not like appendicitis. When you cut away the appendix, the problem is gone. Your back pain is due to anatomical changes as a result of years and years of wear and tear. You did not feel it until recently, but it has been brewing in your body for the past few decades. The treatments you receive here can only make you feel better, but I cannot reverse the arthritic changes you have. Our goal is to make your pain more manageable, but to take it away completely is often unrealistic."

"What did you mean? Are you saying that I have this pain because I am old?" Carol frowned. "I have so much energy and I feel so young. My health and my body have been doing very well. I cannot accept this kind of pain, no matter what you say. Is there anything to get rid of it completely? Can I have surgery to cure it?"

"Surgery can alleviate the pain related to the nerve root impingement," I explained, "but surgery can not cure age-related degenerative changes. Even though it is difficult to deal with this situation on a chronic basis, Carol, you need to make a decision based on realistic expectations."

Unsurprisingly, Carol saw a few spine surgeons, and as expected, nobody could promise her that she would have a pain-free spine after surgery. When she came back to see me, she announced her decision.

"I decided that I don't want surgery. All the doctors seem to be useless, according to what I heard from them. If they can't cure me, what is the surgery good for?"

For that question, I had no answer.

Carol stayed with me for a while longer to receive more treatments. Inevitably, she was dissatisfied with the results. She had no problems with daily activities and her discomfort was quite minimal. However, she complained bitterly about how she was unable to keep up with her highly competitive, professional-level tennis games.

Carol was far from being alone, feeling dejected from not being in perfect shape. I have seen many patients in their seventies, eighties, and even nineties who try awfully hard to live an active lifestyle. What can be more beautiful for me, than to witness energy and happiness during the advancing years of these patients?

However, everything we do has a downside. While my patients strive to remain youthful, some have difficulty accepting the reality of aging, as if aging is not a natural path in life, but a shameful state to be in.

In fact, the International Narcotics Control Board revealed that Americans use far more opioids to deal with the natural effects of aging than any other country in the world. As Keith Humphreys, a professor of psychiatry at Stanford University points out: "For many complicated reasons, cultural factors may tend to increase U.S. opioid consumption."[23]

Humphreys describes:" for example, a fifty-five-year-old may feel acute back and leg pain after doing the workout that was easy when he was twenty-five. A European who finds himself in this situation might reflect sadly that aging must be accepted as part of life, but the achy American might demand that his doctor attend to what he or she believes is a fixable problem."

Everyone gets wrinkles on his or her face, no matter what. Even the most expensive cream or the best surgeon cannot make a person look like twenty-one forever. Our bodies, our bones, ligaments, muscles, and tissues all get older. Just like wrinkles, everyone hates them, but they are inevitable.

Rather than constantly being bothered by the inevitable, however, we can choose to accept each wrinkle as a beautiful memory. We can marvel at the essence and beauty special to each decade of our lives. We can and should always, at every age, to live our lives to the fullest. We, however, do not have to do everything we did at twenty, when we are sixty, or eighty. In fact, it is important to learn about the physiological changes of aging and accept our age, along with all the degenerative joints, and the pains and aches accompanying with advancing age, in order to stay healthy, avoid injuries, and make the most of what we have.

Eventually, Carol and I talked about the reality of her life. She is a very intelligent woman and ultimately recognized that brain activity could surpass her need to slam a ball across a court. Carol didn't give up tennis and I'm happy to know that she still plays doubles, just to maintain her physical shape. She also became a whiz at the card game of Bridge. It was just a matter of adjustment, and she is still playing to win a different game, in which she can feel comfortable.

---

23   https://www.aspeninstitute.org/wp-content/uploads/2018/01/AHSG-Final-Report-2017_compressed-2.pdf

Long March to Normalcy

BACK PAIN OF all types is a common condition that may have a tremendous impact on a patient's life. Low back pain is and always has been a worldwide problem. Prevalence of low back pain increases with age, so it is only expected that there is an increasing rate of pain as people live longer and the population grows older.

Considering the significant increase in the prevalence of back pain over time, it is understandable that there are similar trends in increasing rates of surgeries to treat it.

Sometimes surgery fails to provide relief or provides only temporary relief of the patient's pain. The International Association for the Study of Pain defines failed back surgery syndrome (FBSS) as "lumbar spinal pain of unknown origin either persisting despite surgical intervention or appearing after surgical intervention for spinal pain originally in the same topographical location."[24]

FBSS occurs with conservative estimates at 20 percent, while other estimates of failure are as high as 40 percent.

The recurrence of pain following surgery may be caused by a multitude of reasons.

Back surgery can bring about mechanical changes within the spinal column, affecting the balance within adjacent structures. This can accelerate degenerative changes in the areas of the spine both above and below the surgical site.

Many patients undergo surgeries to make space for nerve root impingement to relieve pain. Just like one gets a scar on the skin when there is a cut, scar tissue may form after the surgical trauma. Gradually taking up the newly freed space, scar tissue can result in spinal stenosis or nerve root impingement again. Even for patients who gain perfect results from their back surgeries, over time, pain may come from completely unrelated new spine problems.

---

24   Baber Z, Erdek MA. Failed back surgery syndrome: current perspectives. J Pain Res. 2016;9:979-987. [PMC free article] [PubMed

Most of my patients come to a pain management office, like mine for spine-related pain; the majority of them being low back pain. Some of them have already had back surgeries.

When Patricia came to my office, she already had two spine surgeries. Patricia was a policewoman in her late forties. Her patrol car spun out and hit the roadside guard rail during one of her highway chases on duty. The car crash left her with a right foot drop and searing pain from her low back down her legs on both sides.

These were typical symptoms of acute lumbar disc herniation pressing on spinal nerves. The foot drop signified severe nerve damage. Patricia had no choice but to undergo surgery to relieve the pressure on her nerve to avoid further deterioration. After the first surgery, the foot drop was gone, and she was able to walk well again.

The pain itself though, returned in full force after a brief period of improvement. Hoping to go back to work in her patrol car, Patricia took the leap of faith and chose to have another spine surgery. Unfortunately, her pain never improved enough for her to work in uniform again. She was deemed disabled and was forced to retire from the police force.

The misfortune of being disabled in her early forties with chronic pain didn't seem to bring Patricia down. Even though she no longer worked as a police officer, she kept her hair short and her voice loud. She was straightforward and no-nonsense. She remained upbeat and buoyant.

"I am still young, Doctor Shue. I want to make the most out of what I have. I understand my limitations, but I would like to go back to walking, exercising, and living a life with as much normalcy as possible."

Patricia had failed back surgery syndrome (FBSS) and this could be a tough problem to treat.

Similar to other pain problems, management for the failed back surgery syndrome includes conservative treatments, steroid injections, and surgery.

Physical therapy and medication management are the cornerstones of first-line pain management. Physical therapy can help patients optimize gait, improve muscle strength and flexibility.

Oral medication includes non-steroidal anti-inflammatory drugs, oral steroids, antidepressants, and opioids. Anti-epileptics such as Gabapentin and Pregabalin can be used to treat neuropathic pain from nerve damage or irritation.

Chronic opioid therapy for non-cancer pain is associated with an increased opioid tolerance and dependence but does not reliably improve long-term relief. Therefore, we try to avoid opioid use.

Interventional pain management, steroid injections, and other minimally invasive procedures have been particularly important tools for doctors to manage pain for patients like Patricia. These patients' symptoms likely come from multiple pain sources. It's important for each patient to be evaluated individually and re-assessed frequently to ensure the most effective treatments are being used to take care of the most significant problems at any given time.

According to Patricia's description of the pain, physical examination, and MRI results, her low back and leg pain were likely to be from a combination of nerve root irritation resulting in radicular pain, and lumbar facet joint arthritis.

Radicular pain, also known as sciatica, is a type of pain that radiates from low back into the legs along the course of a spinal nerve root. It is caused by compression, inflammation and injury to a spinal nerve root, resulting from a herniated disc, spinal stenosis, and scar tissues around the nerve exit points. Leg pain can be accompanied by numbness, tingling, muscle weakness, and loss of reflexes.

For Patricia, the radicular pain that shot down her leg was most consistent with spinal nerve irritation, probably from surgical scar tissues. The most appropriate treatment option for this pain would be epidural steroid injections (ESIs).

ESIs are the most commonly performed procedure in pain clinics around the world. ESI can be a useful tool for both treating the symptoms of radicular pain after surgery and preventing or delaying the need for surgery. A meta-analysis, published in Pain Physician in 2014, suggests that between one-third and one-half of patients considering surgery for spinal pain can avoid it in the short term with ESI[25].

Additionally, facet joint arthritis was most likely responsible for Patricia's stiffness and the band-like deep achy pain across her low back. Facet joints are small joints along the two sides of the vertebral column, connecting the vertebral bodies along the spine. They are essential to allow the low back to twist and turn.

From wear and tear over time, or from traumatic surgical stress, arthritis forms in the facet joints. When this happens, every time the back is turned or twisted, which is constantly happening in everyone's daily life, the joints are irritated, resulting in pain and stiffness. For this problem, treating the small nerves innervating the facet joints, called medial branches, with steroid injections produce the best results.

Patricia listened intently to each of her options. Her medical records indicated that she had tried most of the choices before her surgeries.

"Patricia, I know that none of these medications, physical therapy, injections, or procedures worked well for you in the past. That was why you had to have surgery. However, your anatomy has changed since your last procedure. It is worthwhile to give these treatment options another chance."

25   https://brieflands.com/articles/aapm-17455.html

"I am all for it. Anything that can make me better, I am willing to try."

I admired this woman for her determination. We decided to keep her on most of her medication, including an NSAID, a neuropathic agent and a muscle relaxant, but less opioids. Patricia had been taking the oxycodone provided by her previous physician. The plan was to taper the opioids down once she obtained some relief from interventional pain management procedures.

I sent her for physical therapy treatments to strengthen her core muscles and improve her flexibility which would both be essential for optimization of her pain management. We also arranged for Patricia to come in for injections.

Patricia responded positively to the injections. An epidural steroid treatment provided about 55 percent relief for the radicular pain in her right leg. A medial branch block with steroids and lidocaine also took away about 85 percent of her pain and stiffness across her low back caused by facet joint arthritis. With this treatment, she was able to further reduce her use of opioids. Life still wasn't perfect, but along with medication, Patricia was able to manage her pain and went about her daily business without too much difficulty.

Chronic pain has a mind of its own. Sometimes it gets worse because the patient has lifted a heavy piece of furniture or played too much golf. Most of the time, it gets worse without any rhyme or reason. It can also get better without treatment. In cases where it doesn't get better, then it's time to consider further treatment.

That was what Patricia had to do. She would come to my office every month for her opioid prescription adjustment. Every four to six months, her pain would become worse. Then she would get an epidural steroid injection or a medial branch block injection, depending on what was bothering her more.

With time, because of Patricia's multiple pain sources, she was getting more steroid injections than I would normally choose to offer. Patricia was young but she was a Caucasian woman, which means she had a high risk to develop osteopenia and osteoporosis as she grew older. Frequent use of steroids is associated with higher risk of bone loss.

To reduce the total amount of steroid use, instead of medial branch block, I changed the treatment for her facet-related pain to radio frequency ablation of the medial branch nerves.

Radio frequency ablation has gained popularity in the past decade as a treatment method for chronic pain patients. This treatment is often used to provide sustained relief if doctors are able to identify which nerve or nerves are responsible for a patient's pain. In Patricia's case, her main source of pain relief came from the medial branch nerve block procedure, which indicated that those small nerves were responsible for her low back pain.

During a radio frequency ablation, thin needles are placed in the same areas targeting the small medial branch nerves responsible for her problem, identified by previous injections. These are special needles. Instead of injecting steroids through the needles, they are connected to a machine. This machine will heat the tips of the needles. Since these needle tips are in close proximity of the small nerves, the nerves would be "burned" and therefore quieted down and will send less effective pain signals to the brain. This is how relief is achieved.

Radio frequency ablation can be used to create lesions in different locations, such as the facet joints, sacroiliac joints, and some peripheral nerves. By controlling the temperature and time of the ablation, this technique can provide various desirable lesion size and therefore specific pain relief.

This treatment can provide relief for three to six months and sometimes longer. Another distinctive advantage of this treatment is that it does not involve the use of steroids. Patients with diabetes or osteoporosis would have less worry about side effects of raised blood sugar, or further loss of bone density under these conditions.

As time went by, Patricia and I became friends. One January morning, she came for her regular follow up appointment.

"I've got something for you."

Patricia winked at me and pulled out her purse. She took out a plastic card and handed it to me. It was the legendary police friends and family card. On the back of the card, it was designated to Dr. Sabrina Shue, and signed by Officer Patricia.

"Put this card right next to your driver's license. If you get pulled over by police, when you take out your driver's license, show them this card. It may help you."

That made my day. Not that I had a free pass to be reckless on the road with this little plastic card, but to be included in a patient's friends and family circle, to me, was an honor and an appreciation of my work.

From then on, every January, without fail, Patricia always gave me a new card, each card was printed with the year, which made it good for those twelve months.

"Don't throw any of them away though," Patricia explained. "Keep them all together next to your driver's license. When you open your wallet, any cop who stops you will see all of your cards lined up together and you will be in good shape."

She laughed and winked at me again, flashing her wallet with a roll of credit cards, demonstrating to me how I should safely use her cards to my best advantage.

After I collected the third card from her, things took a turn for the worse for Patricia. Her car was rear-ended when she was at a full stop at a red traffic light. The new lumbar spine MRI and other imaging studies did not indicate any major changes, but Patricia's pain became much worse, once again. Her surgeon, however, did not think any further operation should be attempted. The pain remained across her low back, radiating down her right leg in the same pattern as before the car accident. The major difference was that the injections which used to help her, stop working.

We looked at other sources to explain Patricia's symptoms, but it was a frustrating process. We tried to treat her sacroiliac joints which could give similar symptoms. No relief. We tried trigger point injections to treat muscle spasms in the back, but they did not help either.

It can be challenging to treat low back pain, as it is, because the symptoms can be from a combination of problems. For patients who had lumbar spine surgeries in the past, it can be more difficult, because the normal anatomy has been significantly altered. Scar formation is a natural part of tissue healing after any surgery. Often, spine surgery will result in the formation of scar tissue within the epidural space. This scar tissue may cause back and leg pain on their own by compressing nerve roots.

In addition, scar tissue may contribute to, or compromise the efficacy of treatments including epidural steroid injections, by preventing the steroid from flowing to and acting on its intended target. These scar tissues, called adhesions, can theoretically be removed, thereby improving baseline pain and drug delivery of epidural injections.

Removal of adhesions typically occurs by delivering hyaluronic acid with hypertonic saline into the epidural space. This works by both mechanical expansion of the space with the volume of medication injected, and by the dissolving of the adhesions.

We finally tried a reduction of adhesion treatment, hoping to release some adhesive tissues in the spine from her previous surgeries, and therefore reducing the impingement and irritation of her nerves. But her pain remained.

Patricia fell back to taking more opioids. This was not a good trend at all. I sat down with Patricia again to discuss her options. With the ineffectiveness of interventional pain management treatments and persistent discomfort, it was time for Patricia to consider spinal cord stimulation therapy.

I explained to Patricia, "The very simplified version of how this device works is this: Imagine you have pain in your knees. You would feel better if you massaged your knees with your hands. That is because your brain gets distracted by the massage. Think of this device as something that can send an electrical signal to your spinal cord and therefore your brain is distracted. You would feel tingling in the area where your usual pain is located. That tingling sensation likely feels much more pleasant to you than the persistent pain.

"That is how you feel relief. It is a very sophisticated device. You will have a remote control, just like a cell phone. You can set programs for different activities because your pain is likely to be different depending on what you do. You can turn it on or off anytime."

Patricia smiled at the very thought of a tingling type of relief.

Since the approval of spinal cord stimulation therapy by the U.S. Food and drug Administration in 1989, the technology has much changed and improved. In 2015, the U.S. FDA approved high frequency spinal cord stimulation therapy which, among other benefits, can provide pain relief without patients feeling the tingling sensations from the stimulator.

Spinal cord stimulation (SCS) is a treatment modality that has shown tremendous potential in the management of failed back surgery pain syndrome. Although the initial cost for SCS placement is not inexpensive, due to the expense of the device and surgical implant procedure, the authors in the PRECISE Study published in 2015, concluded that SCS implantation would be cost-effective when taking into consideration of savings due to the improvement of quality of life in a long run[26].

This study underscores the continued costs of untreated spinal pain on society as a whole, including loss of productivity, costs associated with disability, emergency room visits, imaging costs, and costs of medication and hospitalizations.

"What do I need to do if I am interested. Where is it done? Is this a surgery?" Patricia asked.

"There are a few steps in the process of getting a Spinal Cord Stimulator." I explained. "First, you will need to get a clearance from a psychiatrist or a psychologist, mainly to make sure you understand the process and have the capacity to operate the device. Then, after insurance approves the therapy, you will come to my office for a trial.

"When you're under light sedation, I will place two leads like two strands of angel hair pasta in the space right outside the spinal cord. This is similar to the epidural steroid injections you had in the past. Under X-ray guidance, I will place two needles in the epidural space, one on each side of the low back. The two leads will be threaded in through the needles. We will wake you up to test if the tingling sensation produced by the devices would cover the painful area in your back and leg. If not, we readjust the leads.

"If it covers the area well, we will then remove the needle and leave the leads inside. I will tape the battery outside on your back. Then you will go home to try it out for about five to seven days. At the end of the trial, I will remove your trial leads in my office. Don't worry," I comforted her, "This only takes a few seconds.

---

26   https://pubmed.ncbi.nlm.nih.gov/25879722/

"During the trial, if your pain is 50 percent or more improved, you are then a candidate for the implant. If you decide to have the implant, I will send you to a spine surgeon to put in the device. The implant will be a surgical procedure in the hospital. It typically takes one to two hours. The advantage of the spinal cord stimulator is that you can try it first in my office as I explained it, without committing to it."

We went over the pros, cons, and alternatives to the spinal cord stimulation therapy. I sent Patricia home with some informational pamphlets and a DVD. I told her if she would like to talk to any of my patients who had the device implanted, I could arrange that for her. After all, having a foreign object inserted into one's body is a concept any patient has to take time to digest and consider.

Before she returned for her next appointment, Patricia called me. "I am ready to go for the stimulator trial. In my situation where nothing else has worked for me so far, I got nothing to lose. I want to enjoy living my life again."

Patricia's spinal cord stimulator trial went smoothly. She received about 70 percent pain relief. Within a month, she had the implant placed in her back.

Overall, like any other medical treatment, patients have a varying degree of response to the spinal stimulator implant therapy. I witnessed patients who obtained almost a hundred percent relief and no longer needed any medication. I had patients who were able to get only mild to moderate pain relief and still needed steroid injections from time to time, while also relying on medication. Some patients were not able to feel better during the trial period and never proceeded to the implant.

Patricia was somewhere in the middle of the spectrum. She still needed a small amount of medication, but she was able to walk, exercise, and live her life, as she put it.

One afternoon, she came for a follow-up appointment. Unlike her usual self, her face was sullen. There were no jolly remarks or winking of her eyes.

"Patricia, is everything okay with you?" I was concerned.

"No." Before she could say more, Patricia started weeping.

I had seen my share of patients cry in my office. But this was completely unexpected. It was just not in Patricia's character to bawl uncontrollably like this in public.

I scrambled and produced a few sheets of tissue for her. Now, I was really worried. Something terrible must have happened. I waited for her to calm down.

"Tomorrow is my birthday. I am turning fifty. I planned this celebration a long time ago. I even bought tickets for a show for my husband and me, and booked a nice restaurant before the show for us. This morning my husband told me he completely forgot about my birthday, and he had a game to go with his buddy tomorrow night.

"It's my fiftieth birthday, for heaven's sake! That damned bastard. I can't believe he is spending the day with a friend instead of me." Patricia's sobbing became louder and louder.

I watched her in awe. I could hardly believe this was the same person I had come to know, or thought I knew, in the past three years. The happy, straightforward, no nonsense ex-cop dissolved into a sea of tears. I quickly realized that I had made the mistake of profiling. Patricia was an ex-cop, but she was a wife and a woman too.

On one hand, I was relieved that nothing terrible had happened. On the other hand, as a woman, I wish I could give a good scolding to her husband and make him spend the special day with her.

Two months went by before Patricia came back to my office. This time it was with a piece of really bad news.

"We just found out that my husband has end-stage liver cancer. The doctors gave him six months to live."

Patricia looked resolved and composed.

"We are preparing for the worst," she said in her straightforward style, "but we are hoping that we could drive together to Nashville, Tennessee. We always wanted to go there, but never had the chance to visit. First, it was because of my job, then my injuries, then my recovery. Now, we are running out of time. But we will work with his doctors and try to make this trip together before the end comes."

Her eyes twinkled a little before she continued.

"You see, I married him late in life. It was a second marriage for both of us. He has grown children and we decided not to have any kids of our own. Because of hardships I couldn't handle as a young woman, I left my parents' house at age eighteen and never went back. Now he's the only family I've got."

My heart ached for Patricia. I still remembered how she sobbed and complained about her husband two months ago. In the face of life and death, everything else became insignificant.

She had been through enough already. I embraced her and wished her luck.

Patricia did not have much luck. In the next few months, her husband quickly deteriorated. They never had the chance to get in a car to drive anywhere but back and forth to the hospital.

After his passing, his adult children would not help with funeral expenses, but gave Patricia lots of trouble regarding the execution of the will. Then Patricia herself was in and out of the hospital again and again. She underwent surgery on her ankle for a chronic condition that also resulted from the car accident as a policewoman. It was supposed to be a simple surgery, but she contracted MRSA in the hospital, an infection resistant to many antibiotics. She had to have a few more operations within a short period of time.

In late December, Patricia came to see me again. The past twelve months seemed to have turned her world upside down. I opened the door to the consultation room, worried and not sure what kind of trouble I would face this time.

Patricia was sitting, looking up at me, smiling. She had an ocean blue blouse on, with matching blue eye liner, which made her pale blue eyes extra bright. Her hair was still short, and a pretty champagne blonde color.

"You look great. How are you?" I was happy to see her in good spirits. I wondered about her resilience and how she had bounced back from her seemingly endless ordeal.

"I feel good. Thank you." Patricia updated me right away. "I have been through enough grief this year to last me a lifetime. I need to do something for myself to make me happy. I am exercising and doing the right things for my health again. I feel good. I visited my best friend in Florida two weeks ago, and I have decided to move down there. There is nothing left in New York for me. I am going to start everything new, and I am really looking forward to it."

Before she left, Patricia said, "I am not sure when I am moving; it might be within the month. But, if I am still around in January, surely, I will bring one of my cards for you." She winked at me, the way she always did and laughed as she left the office.

January came and went. I never saw Patricia again. I thought of her often, imagining how she was starting her new life in sunny Florida, with her best friend beside her, sipping a cool drink at the beach. I never got my fourth card from Patricia, but I was happy for her.

On a beautiful spring day, one of my staff members came to my office and brought me the news. "Someone called the office and said she was a member of Patricia's family. She wanted to let you know that Patricia passed away about a month ago. She was taken to the ER but died there. I asked her what Patricia died from, but all she said was it was a sudden death. She had no further information."

"Live Each Day Like It's Your Last." This slogan is seen often. But how should we live, given that life is short, and time is forever running out on us?

Generations of scholars and sages have dwelled on this question, from the Chinese philosopher Lao Tzu to the medieval theologian Venerable Bede, from the Renaissance essayist Michel de Montaigne to the anthropologist Ernest Becker.

I don't have an answer. However, Patricia seemed to have helped me understand it all a little better. All three police friends and family cards have long expired and no longer carry any weight for their intended purpose.

I still keep all three in my wallet, along with my driver's license, exactly as Patricia told me to do. I have yet needed to flash them out to any police officers, knock on wood. Every time I open my wallet, I see the cards. They remind me of the pale blue eyes full of optimism and resilience. They remind me to appreciate today, the day that I am enjoying, right now, right at this moment.

When Things Go Wrong: And They Do

AARON, ONE OF my youngest patients, was involved in an automobile accident where his body was thrown toward the left and his head banged on the driver's side window. He immediately developed wretched pain in his neck.

Being a healthy young man in his twenties, he brushed it off and thought everything would get better on its own. Instead of going to an Emergency Department in a nearby hospital, he didn't give further thoughts to his symptoms.

In the next few weeks, however, he started having unremitting pain in his neck, which would radiate from the center in the back of his neck down to the shoulders, arms, forearms, and hands. Occasionally, he felt as if water was running down his arms, or bugs crawling over his shoulders. His hands would get numb and twitch on their own from time to time, without any reason.

Shortly after the accident, Aaron went to work in the IT business. Working on the computer all day and sitting in an upright position at his desk became torturous. He started taking all kinds of medication to quiet down his pain so that he could keep up with his demanding job. It took a full year after his car accident for Aaron to come to my office, because his best friend told him about me.

When I entered the consultation room, he reached out to shake my hand.

"Hey, Dr. Shue. I knew you'd figure out a way to get rid of this pain because my friend, Gary told me everything about what you do.

"I have tried all kinds of anti-inflammatory medication, Advil, Aleve, prescription strength NSAIDs that my other doctors gave me, Tylenol, and muscle relaxants. I also tried exercises, physical therapy, chiropractic treatments and that was prescribed by my primary care doc. And before you say anything about that, I already know it is not good to be on opioids, but that is the only way I can work. I am only in my twenties, but most of the time, I feel like I'm a hundred years old."

Aaron was depressed and exhausted, and his struggle wore me out as I listened to what he had been through.

His medical records indicated that his neck MRI showed multiple disc herniations. A disc is the soft spongy material that sits between two cervical vertebrae and acts as a shock absorber in the cervical spine.

There are six cervical discs, which absorb the majority of the impact to the spine and enable the neck to handle various stresses and loads. With the trauma of a car accident, a disc's soft center can push through a small crack in the disc's exterior tough layer, resulting in a bulging or herniated disc, pinging, and irritating the surrounding nerves.

Some people don't experience symptoms, but others may have neck and arm pain, as well as tingling, numbness, or weakness in the affected area. The herniated discs and pinched nerves explained why Aaron had pain in his neck and those weird sensations in his arms and shoulders.

"Aaron, it looks like you have tried all reasonable conservative treatments without much relief. Has anyone talked to you about an epidural steroid injection for your neck and arm pain?" I asked.

"Yes, but I am scared to death about injections. I can't imagine letting anyone stick a needle in my neck. I heard that people sometimes get paralyzed by it. You don't know how long it took for my friend to convince me to come here. I guess the pain finally took over and I am just desperate," Aaron answered truthfully.

I understood Aaron's fear which is shared by many of my patients. The injection is called an "epidural" injection because the medication is given in a location called the epidural space. It is an area between the spinal canal wall and the dura matter, which is the protective sheath that encloses the spinal cord and spinal fluids. The epidural space runs from the top of the neck all the way to the bottom of the low back.

Since all spinal nerves pass through the epidural space before they reach our arms, legs, and other parts of the body, medication given in the epidural space would reach and work on spinal nerves, calm down the ones irritated by disc herniations and improve the discomfort.

The epidural space is usually between 4mm to 7mm wide, the neck being the narrowest part. If the needle goes too far and pokes a hole in the dura matter—the protective sheath of the spinal cord—spinal fluid may leak out, resulting in a spinal headache. A spinal headache can last a few days, requiring the patient to lie flat during that period of time. If the patient sits upright, the headache gets much worse because the brain is being pulled down by gravity without the normal amount of spinal fluid around the brain that acts like a cushion.

If a spinal headache is annoying, then a spinal cord injury is the most dreaded. If the needle goes in even further and pierces the spinal cord, permanent injury can occur, which does have the potential to result in paralysis. However, the entire procedure is done under constant X-ray guidance in a delicate and precise manner.

I told Aaron that I would numb the skin on his neck, place the needle, and advance it very slowly and carefully. I always check the picture with every step until the needle tip is close to the epidural space. Then I use a special syringe and technique to locate the space. I confirm the needle is in the right spot by using a small amount of contrast fluid which shows up on the screen.

"We only give you the medication when we are certain that the needle is correctly situated," I told Aaron. "The most important thing you need to do while I am working is to stay very still and not make any sudden movements during the procedure, because the margin of error is only a few millimeters.

"Believe or not, this procedure is very well tolerated by patients. The area that the needle has to travel to get to the epidural space actually is not sensitive. Patients are not significantly bothered by the procedure.

"The injections, however, do carry risks. We do not recommend any injections to people who have not tried other non-invasive treatments. It is an analysis of the potential benefit and pain relief you can get from the injection versus the potential risks. But if your pain is interfering with your life and well-being to a certain threshold, then it is time to consider the injection.

"This threshold is different for everyone," I continued to explain. "You are the one experiencing it and will be the one having the procedure. We can help you make your decision, but you are the ultimate decision maker. Every patient responds to medical treatments differently. You have a particularly good chance to feel better. However, nobody knows how much better you will feel, or for how long.

"Overall, epidural injections are very safe when done appropriately. It is like driving a car. All kinds of terrible things can happen when we drive, but we still feel comfortable driving every day because overall it is very safe to do."

I proceeded to talk to Aaron regarding the importance of him going back to exercises, and making some significant work environment changes, such as getting ergonomically sound office furniture, and taking frequent breaks to stretch while working with his computer. I also discussed my concern about the risk of using opioids on a long-term basis. We both agreed that it was time to do something else to relieve his discomfort so that he could get off the narcotics.

A few days later, Aaron made an appointment for the cervical epidural steroid injection. It went very smoothly. When he came back for a follow-up visit a month later, he looked elated.

"The tingling and strange sensation in my arms are mostly gone," he said, "but I still have this pain and tightness in the left side of my neck, going to the top of my left shoulder. Maybe I did not pay too much attention to it before because my other pain consumed my mind. Now, every time I turn my head, I feel like I can hear my neck grinding and crackling on the left side. Is that even possible or am I going crazy?"

I laughed and shook my head. "No, Aaron. You are far from crazy. What you just described is real."

Then I examined Aaron again and found that he had tenderness along left side of his neck, which was made worse when he turned and tilted his head upward. It seemed to me that Aaron had facet joint-related pain in his neck.

Facet joints are the small joints on each side of the spine linking the vertebrae together. These small joints allow us to turn our neck and twist our low back. This means that the facet joints are in constant motion every day. Just like the knee or hip joints, facet joints can get significant wear and tear over time, resulting in arthritis. Additionally, trauma such as a whiplash injury to the neck from the car accident he had can irritate the facet joints.

Although facet syndrome is most often associated with age-related degenerative changes, young people like Aaron, who have had a traumatic event can also have significant pain from facet joint irritation and inflammation. Treatment approach for addressing facet joint pain is the same, regardless of whether the condition resulted from routine wear and tear or a traumatic injury.

"Aaron, the little joints on the left side of your neck are probably irritated and inflamed. They can give you pain with neck movements. The trauma from the car accident can accelerate the development of arthritis in the facet joints and give you that grinding and crackling sensation when you turn your head. You can try medication, exercises and give it some time to calm down. If the pain is severe, we can quiet it by injecting some medication targeting the medial branch nerves, which are small nerves controlling the facet joints."

"Let me have the injection, Dr. Shue. The epidural was really not as bad as I thought it would be. I only regretted that I did not have it done sooner and that I suffered so long. I have tried other things throughout this year. Now, I just want to get better."

It did not take long for Aaron to make his decision, after we, again went over the pros, cons, and alternatives of different treatment options. Within a month, he returned and had the medical branch block as the treatment for his left-sided facet joint related neck pain. The combination of this treatment and the previous epidural steroid injection finally took away the majority of Aaron's pain.

"Now your pain is reduced, but your neck is never going to be the same as what it was before the car accident. Remember to do stretching and strengthening exercises that you learned from your physical therapist every single day. Strong muscles and good flexibility will keep you from having to come back. Even though we will always be happy to see you, I am sure you won't be thrilled if you have to come too frequently. Remember: In this case, less is more."

I sent Aaron off with happiness about his success. By that time, he already weaned himself off oxycodone and only was taking ibuprofen and Tylenol as needed.

Over a three-year period, Aaron would come once or twice a year for treatment for his neck pain. Overall, his discomfort was mild and manageable. He would have episodes of worsened pain especially if he had to work overtime with his endless projects and deadlines. These problems pushed his exercise routine to the bottom of his priority list. Despite his pain, he remained off opioids for which both of us were happy.

It was a perfect day in June when everything appeared to be lovely outside as well as in the office. I was happy to see everyone, albeit the fact that the waiting room was packed with new and old patients. Aaron was with us for a medial branch block for his left-sided neck pain again.

By this time, he was an office veteran. He and my staff members all knew each other very well and enjoyed the time together.

He climbed up the procedure table and lay down on his right side, so that his left side of the neck was facing up for the procedure. Under X-Ray guidance, I inserted two thin needles in place and injected half a millimeter of medication mixture in each of the two locations.

As I was pulling the needles out, making small talk, Aaron's whole body tensed up, and he screamed, "Something is wrong! Something is wrong! I can't see! My eyes can't see!"

"What?" I felt my blood run cold and thought, "Did he just go blind?"

"Turn him on his back and check his vital signs," I told my nurse.

The staff member and I immediately turned Aaron on his back. I surveyed his vital functions. He was breathing, had a good pulse, oxygen level, and blood pressure. He was waving his right hand over his eyes, as he stared into space.

"I can't see my hands. I can't see," Aaron kept screaming.

"What just happened?"

My heart was racing, and I started having cold sweats. As Aaron seemed to be stable in terms of his vital signs, I quickly examined each step of the procedure in my head. There was no blood on aspiration when I double-checked the needles before I gave the medication. That meant the needles were not in any blood vessels. I quickly looked over the X-ray image on the screen which showed all needles in perfect spots on bony structures. I was certain everything was done to my satisfaction during Aaron's procedure.

Oh, no! Could he have had an optic nerve ischemia? Or a stroke?

Fear struck me with such a powerful force, I was afraid I would faint. I thought of these extremely rare, but much dreaded complications for interventional pain management doctors. I wondered if this worst nightmare had happened to Aaron at this very moment.

During neck injections, the needle tip comes into close proximity with some important structures including the vertebral artery and some small arteries supplying the spinal cord. If a needle is placed by accident into the vertebral artery or other blood vessels, the volume or the content of the medication mixture can cause vertebral artery dissection, or microvascular embolization, which means small medication particles going in small blood vessels resulting in their constriction. These can potentially alter normal blood flood into the brain, causing a stroke. If normal blood going to the eye was interrupted, the patient would have blindness due to optic nerve ischemia. If Aaron had gone blind, I did not want to think about what would happen. He came in a young, healthy, able person, contributing positively to the society. Imagine the pain and suffering he would have to endure for the rest of his long life? In this case, even though every step of the injection was done properly according to the standard of care, things still had gone terribly wrong.

I never lifted my eyes off Aaron. He was breathing well, moving his facial muscles and all four limbs well. His speech was perfect.

What is going on? Everything else looks good with Aaron, except his loss of vision.

Aaron had the same procedure multiple times in the past. It could not be an allergic reaction because no new medication was used. The medication mixture that I used did not contain small particles that would potentially cause vasospasm. By this time, it was clear that Aaron was stable, and I needed to get more information from him.

"Aaron, are you not able to see anything at all? Everything is black? When you lost vision, did it happen as if there were a black curtain coming down in front of your eyes?" I asked, anxiously, awaiting his answer.

"It was blurry." He deeply sighed. "I never really lost my vision. It just became blurry. And now I am almost back to normal." He smiled.

Those words were the most beautiful music I had ever heard in my life, and a huge weight was lifted from my shoulders.

Aaron did not go blind. Most importantly, he was already almost back to normal within a few minutes from the onset of the event. "You never lost your vision. You were always able to see even when you yelled that you could not see?" I wanted to avoid any misunderstanding.

"Yes. Sorry, did I scare you? I kind of sensed that you were overly concerned which made me scared too."

"Yes, you scared me. I thought you went blind and completely lost vision which would be a quite different beast to deal with. Along with the lack of other symptoms, I was relieved that you did not have a stroke or any nerve damage."

"Well, you scared me too, so we're even." Aaron was back to his usual self as his blurry vision completely resolved.

"So, what happened? I never experienced this before," he asked.

"Most likely, what happened was that at least one of the two needles was probably placed in a blood vessel. Even though I use multiple ways to check for any possible needle placement in blood vessels during the procedure, sometimes, it can escape all areas of the safety net and still happen. When the numbing medication, Lidocaine, was injected into the blood vessel, it quickly went to the brain. This can lead to symptoms including ringing in the ears, numbness in the tongue and lips, metallic tastes in mouth, dizziness, and as in your case, blurred vision. Because the amount of medication I gave you was small, your symptom was very brief."

Aaron showed a perfect score on his neurological examination and vital signs. I still asked him to stay in the office for an extra hour, just to be sure he was back to his usual state of health before I let him go home.

Complications, like shadows of any and all medical procedures, unfortunately, cannot be completely eliminated. If a procedure is repeated frequently enough, something is bound to happen. It is just a matter of time. Here is the analogy: we cannot stay in the house forever if we are afraid of car accidents; similarly, we cannot stop offering patient treatments if we excessively worry about complications.

As physicians, we try our best to decrease the risk and complications by offering procedures only to patients who would benefit from them. We help patients understand the pros, cons, alternatives, and potential risks of any procedures so they can make the best decisions, choosing the safest medication, while balancing the effectiveness of them. We perfect our technical skills by keeping up with the newest recommendations from the medical societies and peer reviews, providing the best and safest working environment with well-trained supportive staff and state of the art equipment. If complications do happen, and they will, we need to make sure we are ready to handle them.

What Aaron experienced was my first case of this kind in all my years of practice. I have read about this very complication often, but when it really happened, it was an incredibly stressful moment in time, especially it mimicked the symptoms of another disastrous potential complication. I was shaken a bit although happy that everything ended up well. All I wanted to do was to relax for a while.

After work that day, I went for my scheduled dental appointment. To tell you the honest to goodness truth, sitting in a dentist's chair with the drill, sizzling on my molar, was the most relaxing moment of that day for me. There I was, just a patient, free from the responsibility of taking care of another human. I relaxed and fell asleep—in the dental chair.

"You yourself, as much as anybody in the entire universe, deserves your love and affection." — Buddha

Myofascial Pain

NANCY, IN HER fifties, was a very soft-spoken woman. It would be rare for me to meet a patient who was so reserved and timid in my office, or in fact, anywhere. Then I learned why.

Nancy suffered with almost twenty years of chronic pain in her neck and shoulders. She endured constant spasms, stiffness, tingling and numbness in her neck, shoulders, and upper torso. She had trouble turning her neck from side to side. It was so bad she would avoid driving, fearing she would have an accident.

Nothing helped her, Nancy admitted. She stretched, used cold and hot compresses, and took Tylenol and NSAIDS.

"I cry myself to sleep most nights. I sometimes feel that my life is so miserable, I don't know if I want to live at all."

With her quiet demeanor, her eyes started to well up with tears.

"For twenty years you have suffered. Have you seen a doctor about it?" I asked with surprise.

"Not really. I never thought it was a real problem. I believe I have the pain because I did not take care of myself. I should be able to deal with it on my own. I feel like a failure because I cannot get better on my own. I did not think I was worth seeing doctors for my pain," Nancy softly said.

What kind of logic was this? I was bewildered and perplexed listening to Nancy. Evidently, she had lived within her own circle of rationale for years and didn't feel worthy enough to seek help and look for relief.

I had legitimate reasons to worry that she could be a victim of battered wife syndrome or childhood abuse, because she clearly had low self-esteem. I carefully chose my words and asked about her childhood and social situations.

She smiled at me. "I know why you are asking me all these questions. I appreciate it, but I have had a normal and fairly good life. My husband is a nice man. I am the one who is giving myself a hard time.

"A close friend of mine told me about you more than a year ago. I made a couple appointments here in the past but ended up canceling them. I just did not think it was right for me to come. But my pain has really gotten to me, and I decided to see you today."

Nancy had no significant medical history or problems. On physical examination, she had tight muscle bands along her neck, shoulders, and upper back, especially in her trapezius muscles on the tops of her shoulders. When I pressed on the bands, Nancy winced and retracted her body to try to get away from my hand, but still, she did not make a peep.

"Did that hurt?" I asked, realizing that she probably would never volunteer much information like my other patients do.

"It hurt so much when you did that. I felt pain shooting down my arm when you pressed on my shoulder," Nancy admitted.

I told Nancy I believed she suffered from myofascial syndrome, which is a chronic pain disorder. Patients with this condition may experience deep, aching pain in muscles. They may feel tender knots in one or multiple muscles.

Injuries or overuse of muscles can lead to formation of tight and sensitive muscle bands. Pressure on these sensitive points in various parts of the body, called trigger points, cause pain in the muscles and sometimes in seemingly unrelated parts of the body. This is called "referred pain."

Trigger points can be caused by muscle tightness, such as a spot within or near a strained muscle from repetitive motions and poor posture. People who experience stress and anxiety may be more likely to develop trigger points. This is thought to be because these people may be more likely to clench their muscles, a form of repeated strain that leaves muscles susceptible to trigger points.

Treatment for myofascial pain syndrome typically includes medication, trigger point injections, and physical therapy. No conclusive evidence supports using one therapy over another.

Since Nancy already tried years of over the counter NSAIDs, stretching exercises without relief, I suggested that she try a procedure to her neck and shoulders called trigger point injections.

There are a variety of different ways to perform trigger point injections. The commonality of the various techniques is that doctors use a fine needle to insert into the tight muscles where the spasms are. The needle would usually be moved up and down within the muscle. This is called "needling," which is thought to break up spasms and scar tissues present in the muscles. Some doctors do not give any medication but only use "dry needling." Some uses numbing medication (Lidocaine or bupivacaine) to reduce the discomfort from the procedure itself. Others inject a mixture of steroids and numbing medication, aiming to reduce inflammation in the area. All these seem to provide similar results.

Doctors are still trying to figure out exactly what mechanism has resulted in trigger points and how different treatments are helping the problem. Some people think the way needling is beneficial is the same way acupuncture works. The needling and stimulation help the body release endorphin—our natural pain killer made by the body—and therefore, we feel better.

I explained to Nancy that this simple, quick, and safe trigger point injection procedure could make a difference in the way she felt.

"Are you sure I really need the shots?" She hesitated, but finally decided to try.

I set my gloved hand on her shoulder to calm her down before I placed the injections in the top of her shoulders and along her tight muscle on the two sides of her spine in the neck and upper back. Her trapezius muscles on the shoulders twitched as the needle went in the belly of the muscles.

"This is called the twitching reaction which we usually see in moderate and severe cases of myofascial pain syndrome like yours," I explained to Nancy.

After the treatment was complete, Nancy already felt the lessening of the stiffness and pain. She looked unconvinced. Then, with doubt on her face, she slowly and carefully turned her head to one side, a little more, then a little further.

"Oh, my goodness! Look how far I can turn my head now. Even only a minute ago, I could never have dreamed of doing just that," Nancy cried out with joy, tears running down her face. "I thought the pain I had was not real. I thought it was only just in my head."

She kept checking to slowly turn her neck left and right, up, and down, still in disbelief.

"I never thought I was worth being treated for my pain. I believed I should just grin and bear it. Finally, I realize how I should feel. It feels so good to be without the terrible pain that I have had for twenty years."

I was aghast at this response, both in terms of her pain relief, and her realization of her physical condition, and most importantly, her self-worth.

As Nancy contained her emotions, I talked to her at length about her treatment plan.

"Nancy, myofascial pain syndrome is a chronic problem. The most important thing to do for your condition is what you do at home. Gentle and mild exercise can help you relax muscles and gain more energy. When your pain allows, try to walk outside more. Swimming is great if you can get access to a pool. I will also send you to a physical therapist to teach you appropriate exercises. If you are stressed and tense, your muscle spasms will likely get worse. Please find ways to relax. Try massage and meditation. Gardening, yoga, going out with friends can all be helpful. Maintain a healthful diet and get enough sleep. Take care of your body and general health. You can come back to get the same treatment every month for the first few months if you need to. There is no steroid involved. I used only numbing medication so side effects are minimal. You have every reason to seek out ways to feel better and I want you to remember this every time you turn your head."

Nowadays, Nancy periodically comes to me for repeat trigger point injections. She calls them "booster shots." I call it a shot of confidence. She told me that she picked up gardening and started going out with her husband and watching movies with friends. In other words, she was finally enjoying life. She is still timid, but she smiles much more. Her smile was something I valued more than the fact that she moved her neck with more grace and ease.

I was happy to see Nancy's improvement because not everyone is able to obtain good results from medical treatments for myofascial pain syndrome. Some research suggests that this problem may develop into fibromyalgia in some patients over time.

"Relationships are like drugs. They either hurt you or
Give you the best feeling of your life." — Wiz Khalifa

Family Dynamics

FIBROMYALGIA IS A chronic condition that features chronic widespread pain. There are two main schools of thoughts within the medical community regarding this disease entity. Some doctors believe that the brains of people with fibromyalgia become more sensitive to pain signals over time and that is why patients experience extraordinary amount of pain, all over their bodies without pathology to correlate the pain.

Doctors on the other side believe that it is either mainly a psychological disease state, or patients suffer from real organic disease processes, not yet discovered by modern medicine.

No matter which side a doctor is with on this controversy, it is generally agreed that exercise, lifestyle changes, coping mechanism training, and non-opioid medication are the main treatment methods.

The above treatment plan was exactly what I emphasized when I met Ella, a woman in her early forties who suffered with chronic widespread whole-body pain, diagnosed as fibromyalgia. Ella came to me with more than ten years of treatment for fibromyalgia. She was taking the equivalent of 300mg of morphine a day. When I talked to her about focusing on lifestyle and general wellness improvement and reducing the amount of opioids, she promptly agreed without making a fuss like some other patients would do.

"I think you're right. Those pain pills make me constipated and tired all day. Even so, my pain is never gone. I often wonder if they are doing anything for me, but I didn't dare to change my medication because I am afraid that my pain would get worse. If you think I should take less medication and if you help me do that, I will work with you."

Every month, when Ella came in for her appointment, we would take off a morphine pill from her regimen. The process was not smooth. She had times where she doubted the plan and found it difficult to stick to the new medication dosage. With encouragement, Ella was slowly but surely able to keep making small progress. Before we knew it, she was down to taking 150mg morphine each day, half of the amount she was on when she first came to me.

Sabrina Shue

"I have to say now that I am taking less morphine pills, my head is clearer. My pain is a little more than before, but there are no major changes. I am glad that I listened to you."

Ella, a sweet woman, was proud of her progress, but she was unhappy. She told me that she was unemployed, depressed, anxious, lonely, and in chronic pain. Soon, I got a glimpse of what might have influenced and shaped her current life.

One day, Ella brought her elderly mother to the office with her. I reviewed the treatment plan and was about to send the prescription to her pharmacy with one less morphine pill a day. Ella's mother interjected, "Wait a minute, wait a minute. Ella, what is going on? How can you let the doctor give you less pain medication? Your pain is so out of control. Don't you need more?" She turned to me. "Doctor, you can't give Ella less than last month. I am her mother. I watch what she goes through every day. She is in terrible pain, and she needs more pain medication, not less."

We are in the middle of a national opioid crisis. With all the media reports and education, more and more family members are aware and concerned about their loved ones' overuse of opioids. They often would accompany patients to their appointments and encourage patients to taper down opioids. Ella's mom seemed to be on the wrong side of the team and was trying to encourage her daughter to take more opioids.

"I understand your concern," I replied. "But Ella has done really well using other coping methods and non-narcotic medication for her pain. I know she is not pain-free, but she knows how to take care of herself. Large amount of opioids are not recommended for her disease. They may do more harm than good in a long run."

I put the ball back in Ella's court.

I turned to Ella and asked, "Are you ready to go forward with our plan to reduce your morphine pills, just like what you did for the past few months?"

The mother stiffened as I leaned toward her and continued, "I would encourage you to support your daughter's endeavor to taper down her medications, especially when she has accomplished so much in the past few months without any problems."

Ella glanced at me and remained silent. She then gazed at her mother. Slowly, she looked at me again. "Yes, my pain has been really bad. It's been difficult for me to take less pain medication." She stopped to take a deep breath. "But let's stick to our plan."

"Ella, but you are going to get yourself into a lot of trouble," her mother grumbled. She stood up, stepped forward toward me, and bawled, "What if she is in severe pain? What does she do then? She won't be able to get out of bed or take care of herself. Her pain is really bad. You doctors don't even understand what she goes through every day." She turned back to Ella. "Ella,

I am telling you. You are going to lie in bed all day for the whole month ahead, begging for my help because you just don't listen to me."

Ella's mother was dismayed by my plan and her daughter's decision, and she was not going to give up.

I breathed a sigh of relief when the mother and daughter duo got up, left my consultation room, and headed toward the office exit.

Then Ella's mother swerved around. She looked me straight in the eye, and growled, "Fibromyalgia and chronic pain have ruined my daughter's life. You have no idea what you are doing to her." She stomped out of my office and didn't look back.

What (or rather who) had actually ruined Ella's life? Was it fibromyalgia? Or was it something else? What I had observed revealed that the reality was likely much more complicated than that.

"Anxiety is a thin stream of fear trickling through the mind.
If encouraged, it cuts a channel into which all other thoughts are
drained." — Arthur Somers Roche

A DIFFERENT KIND OF PAIN

WHEN I WAS still talking to my patient in a consultation room, I heard a noise coming from the adjacent room, through the wall. It sounded like a strange yelping, almost like a bark.

Who brought a pet in for a doctor's appointment?

Nobody would bring a pet to a doctor's office.

Oh, no! It could not be from a patient. Could it?

I opened the door to the next consultation room. A woman who appeared to be in her late seventies was sitting in the chair, writhing, while making the bark-like sounds I heard. I took a deep breath, sensing this might be a tough case.

It turned out that I was right.

Mabel was only in her early sixties, yet she looked at least ten years older. She'd been through three lumbar spine surgeries, and her spine was somewhat twisted, making her right hip jut out to the side.

For the past five years or so, she was kept on a large dose of opioids. A month before she came to my office, she had ingested too many pain pills and ended up in the hospital.

"I almost died, Dr. Shue. I almost died. I'm so afraid of taking those pills. I don't want to take them anymore because I don't want to die." Mabel started crying, mixing her tears with her unique bark. "But I'm in so much pain. I can't walk, stand, or even sit for any length of time."

I combed through Mabel's history and physical examination. She had a multitude of spine-related issues leading to her severe and persistent low back pain.

Low back pain can come from multiple sources. It's the reason why so many people are affected by this ailment. The complexity of it explains why low back pain is difficult to treat, because every source of pain can mimic another. Diagnosis is not always straightforward and it is often a conundrum for me.

In Mabel's case, her most bothersome pain that day emanated from the two sides of the upper buttocks. She had severe tenderness in that area where one can feel the bony structures. This suggested that she likely had irritation of the sacroiliac joints, which probably contributed to her pain.

The sacroiliac joints connect the two sides of the sacrum, the bottommost part of the spine, to the ilia, which are the largest part of the hip bones in the pelvis. These joints are essential for stabilizing the human body and they allow the lower extremities to bear weight evenly and walk with a good balance. The sacroiliac joints can get loose or arthritic over time. This can cause patients to suffer aggravating discomfort in the low back, upper buttock area, sometimes even shooting around to the groin or down through the legs.

"I can't take this pain anymore. Can't you give me something stronger? My pain pills are doing nothing to me, except for the fact that they almost killed me." Mabel kept weeping.

"Mabel, didn't you just tell me that you almost died after taking too many opioids? If you take that many of them, even if you don't overdose, you may get dizzy, drowsy, have a fall, and severely hurt yourself."

"I know you damn doctors just don't want to give me my pills."

I was caught off guard by her sudden change in attitude.

"Look at you. You're afraid that I'm addicted to them. Just give them to me and let me die. I rather die than live like this," Mabel wailed. "God, please take me now. I don't want to live anymore. Take me now!"

Mabel glared at me and became increasingly hysterical.

I patiently gave her time to calm down.

I then explained to her that, since she had only tried opioids for pain, it would be a good idea to give a chance to interventional pain management injections.

"But, in the past, I tried epidural injections. They never, ever worked," Mabel replied.

"Correct," I answered.

"The epidural injections were aimed to treat your spinal nerve irritation and inflammation in the lumbar spine. You still have that problem. However, you also have pain from the sacroiliac joints. This is frequently seen in patients who have had spine surgeries in the past. Surgical changes can affect the balance of your back and accelerate the process of arthritic changes.

"A steroid injection into the sacroiliac joint is an entirely different treatment, for a separate problem. I think you have a good chance to feel better," I calmly explained.

"Give it to me then. I would do anything to feel better." Mabel was game right away. "Dr. Shue, you're going to give me my shots now, right?"

Many patients would come to my office, expecting an injection during their initial visit. Who can blame them? They're in severe pain and want treatment as soon as possible.

The logistics are complicated. First, we must determine the patient is an appropriate candidate with the correct pathology and indication for an injection. Prior to injections, we need to review MRI or imaging reports, which patients may have forgotten to bring. Some patients cannot have injections unless they have stopped taking certain medications, such as anticoagulants, days in advance prior to the treatment. Often, we have to get permission from their prescribing doctors to hold these essential medication therapies.

Most importantly, we are required to obtain prior authorizations for these procedures. Nowadays, doctors don't get to do what we think are best for our patients. We can only do what insurance companies think are appropriate for their patients. This process, while discounting the importance of individualized healthcare, can also be labor intensive. My staff frequently spend more than an hour on the phone to obtain one prior authorization. This ordeal can be time consuming, taking a few days to a few weeks for the paperwork to be processed, depending on patients' insurances.

Mabel didn't want to hear any of that when I tried to explain that she would have to come back another time for her injection.

"How dare you send me home without making me better today? I cannot live with this pain for another minute. I want to die! I want to die!" She relapsed into a mess of tissues and tears. "I'm not leaving until you do something for me today. Otherwise, you'll find me dead hanging from your office ceiling tomorrow morning!"

I gave in. It would be too difficult to explain, and too much paperwork for me to fill out, if Mabel had hanged herself in my office.

I took her to the procedure room. The injection went smoothly, despite the fact that the entire process was peppered with Mabel's screaming, cursing, and her vocal desire for God to take her.

When I went to check on her in the recovery area, moments later, Mabel looked transformed. "You know what, Dr, Shue, with the injection, I felt a wave of coolness had come down on me. I feel as if my body is encased in a velvet blanket. My pain was lifted off from my chest. Now I can even breathe better."

Her description was rather dramatic. Yet, I found her quietude more striking. I was quite relieved.

"I am so sorry I was nasty toward you early on. I was just in so much agony and I was out of my mind. I apologize," Mabel said softly.

"That's quite all right, Mabel."

I was elated that she looked and felt better.

Patients like Mabel are not strangers to us. Pain can change people's personalities. When people suffer, they can become short-tempered, irritated, snappish, or even downright angry. When patients show up in my office, they, more than likely have gone through multiple health care professionals, including internists, orthopedists, and physical therapists. Many patients didn't know that doctors like us, interventional pain specialists, even existed.

By the time they eventually come to us, they are already exhausted by the unrelenting pain and stress. They're frustrated by the convoluted health care system. Some patients acknowledge that this process is to ensure that they have tried conservative treatments before they are sent to me. However, others are not always as understanding. They take their anger out on me and my office staff. When they come, they scream, act demanding, and are uncooperative.

We sincerely try to be empathetic and accommodating. I warn all new staff members about our unique challenges. To work in a pain management office, compassion and patience are essential.

"How do you handle all your problematic patients? Don't they drive you crazy?" Other doctors and friends ask me this question often, knowing a thing or two about the mayhem that may occur in a pain management suite.

I tell them, "Every time I encounter a difficult patient, I say to myself: Imagine I were a family member, a wife, a daughter, or a mother to this patient, having to deal with him/her every day? How lucky that I am only the doctor. I only have to manage him/her once every few months. Life is good to me."

However, my attitude and my self-comforting tactic didn't work in Mabel's case.

When Mabel got some relief from the sacroiliac joint injection, we decided together that I would decrease her opioids. I encouraged her to use injections instead of an escalated dose of opioids, if her pain should worsen.

Every few months, she would come for another treatment, each time with the same drama, as if an old TV episode were being repeated again and again.

She would call my emergency after-hour number from time to time, usually late at night.

"I am so sorry to bother you. But my pain is so bad. I want to take another pill. I just wanted to call you to make sure it is safe for me to do that. I don't want to overdose again. I don't want to die."

Each time, I would go over what she already took for the day and explain to her that she was still within her safety limit. It would be okay for her to take another pill. I would also tell her what to do next time when she encountered the same situation.

Before long, I realized that no matter how many times I had explained things to her, she would not dare to manage her pills without calling me first. She was severely anxious and needed me to hold her hands and walk her through step by step.

Mabel's calls grew more frequent, particularly at night, as she got more comfortable with me. Sometimes she would call every night for most of the week. It started to feel that I talked to her much more frequently than to any of my own children.

I had to put a stop before this relationship grew more dependent than I had intended. More importantly, Mabel needed professional psychological help to keep her anxiety under control.

I called her internist, as well as her previous psychiatrist. I learned that Mabel was well known for her challenging behavior. She had been a big shot career woman in her younger days. Disability and chronic pain from her spine disease had taken a big toll on her, forcing her to retire and lose contact with most of her friends and colleagues.

Two out of her four children were estranged from her for various reasons. The two daughters who would see her from time to time, lived out of state. Constant pain, anxiety, lack of family support, and early termination of a successful career all pushed her over the edge. Mabel developed severe depression. All of it was exacerbated by her near-death experience with her accidental opioid overdose.

She refused to see any other psychiatrists when her previous one moved away to Florida, because she insisted that she couldn't trust anyone.

Her internist told me, "I'm doing my best to manage her anxiety and depression as I have known her for years, poor woman. But she seems to like you a lot."

I was flattered, but I couldn't tell if that was a blessing or a curse.

Mabel's situation took a turn for the worse when she suffered a fall. She tripped on a rug in her apartment. She did not break any bones, but her pain got much worse. She had new problems in her low back, which differed from the pain associated with her sacroiliac joints.

We repeated imaging studies on her lumbar spine, which did not show any new changes. We tried other steroid injections but did not get good results. She refused to consider other procedures, such as a spinal cord stimulator or a morphine pump, because she was deathly afraid of having any kind of surgery again.

One day, Mabel came, screaming and barking in pain, like déjà vu. "Do something, doctor! Do something! How can you watch me in this terrible condition? Do something! Anything!"

I was running out of options. She was already taking a large amount of opioids and had just received a steroid injection a few weeks before.

Do something. Anything. I thought to myself.

I knew doing nothing would initiate a rerun of a horror movie. I would need to pacify Mabel with something tangible and safe.

"Why don't I do some trigger point injections in your low back. Maybe that would calm down the pain and spasm in your muscles."

A trigger point injection is a procedure where a numbing medication, such as Lidocaine, is injected into areas with muscle spasms. I did not anticipate that it would do much for Mabel. Her problems were much deeper than the muscle layers.

To my surprise, she quieted down after the procedure.

Thenceforward, every few weeks, she would return for the same treatment, reporting to me that she would feel better for a couple of weeks each time.

"I did not expect trigger point injections would help Mabel." I shared my puzzlement with my office manager who wholly agreed.

"I think Mabel just needs to see you and talk to you every few weeks," she said. "Any touch by you would have made her better, no matter what you do. She is just too lonely and too anxious."

What an insight that was.

Chronic pain and anxiety do go hand in hand. They poison each other, making both conditions more severe and harder to treat. For Mabel, every pill she took made her worry about overdosage. If she did not take it, she grew anxious, fearing the terrible pain would come get her at any moment.

She canceled plans with friends because she did not want to make a fool of herself having to leave early, due to her discomfort. Then she sank into depression because she felt lonely.

She looked forward to visits with her grandchildren, only to cancel a trip at the last minute because she thought she looked ridiculous in her condition.

She refused to see family members who asked to visit her for the very same reason. Yet, when nobody came to celebrate holidays with her, Mabel cursed them out for being cold-blooded and ungrateful.

Daily errands became exhausting. She worried whether she had brought enough pills with her. When she carry extra pills, on the other hand, she agonized over the possibility of losing them. She would drop everything and rush home in order to take her next pain pill on time.

Mabel was consumed by her anxiety related to her pain and her pills. Instead of them controlling her pain, her pills had controlled her life.

Mabel's frequent visits to my office didn't free me up from her nighttime phone calls. In fact, the situation got worse. She would call multiple times in one day, even in the middle of the night, or early morning hours when I was busy sending my children off to school.

She would scream in my voice mail recording:

"I want to die. I want to die. I don't want to live. Call me. Dr. Shue!"

"I couldn't find my pills. I am going to withdraw soon. What should I do? Call me now. Call me!"

"I forgot what I took today. I am in so much pain. But I don't dare to take any pills. What should I do? I don't want to die. Could you please call me, right away!"

"I am standing on the balcony. I don't want to live anymore. I want to jump off the building. Will you call me right now?"

I became physically and mentally exhausted dealing with Mabel. By this time, I was pretty sure that Mabel would not harm herself or get in major trouble. She just needed me to call and talk to her. However, I still had to answer her calls right away. It would become a ticking time bomb if I had ignored any calls like these. What if she really did jump this time? How would I live with that?

I could not go on like this, so I sat down with her in my office, door closed.

"Mabel, if you still want me to be your doctor, you need to do these things I'm about to tell you: Go see a psychiatrist for your anxiety. You're having trouble taking care of your own medication needs. You need to hire help at home or go to a nursing home. Let me speak to your children regarding your situation. You should let them help you too. I am your doctor, not your daughter. A lot of your calls at night weren't about medical problems. Call your family and friends first, not me," I stated firmly.

"But my daughters are so busy," Mabel said. "They have their own lives. I don't want to disturb them. They have to work full-time jobs and take care of their children. I cannot bother them."

I felt as if somebody had hit me in my chest and taken my breath away.

"Mabel, I work twelve hours a day and I have three young children to care for. I need to live my life too. You feel bad that you'd have to bother your own daughters, but I also need time to be with my family. If you can't draw the line between our doctor-patient relationship, then you should find another doctor to take care of you."

Mabel became quiet. I sat quietly too. Moments passed. After all, Mabel was a smart and educated woman. She apparently got my point because she stood up and left the office.

After that talk, her phone calls began to slow down. My problem of nighttime disturbance was gone, but Mabel's problems remained. As frustrated as I was that day, I had a soft spot for her in my heart.

I eventually got her permission to speak to her children. I wanted to work together with the family members to convince Mabel to get domestic help, and I called the first number on her chart.

"How can I do anything? She is an able adult," the first daughter I called said. "She can make her own decisions. There is nothing I can do."

The phone call was short and to the point. My heart sank and I began to understand why Mabel didn't want to call her family even when she needed them. It wasn't the first time I encountered elderly patients' children who were disinterested in their parents' healthcare needs. It is a regretful social problem where the younger generation forgets that it is their responsibility as children when their parents become sick and unable to care for themselves.

I moved on to call her older daughter. Luckily, I was able to find some support from her. After months of back-and-forth debates, Mabel finally moved into an assisted living facility.

Through the grapevine, I learned that she remained a difficult patient because of her strong personality and character. However, she finally agreed to see a psychiatrist. She also made some new friends there and began to enjoy more social activities.

Her bothersome conditions were still there, but her anxiety seemed to have reduced. She stopped talking about her fear of dying or her wish to die, and this gave me tremendous relief.

She still showed up with her dramatic entrances when she needed an injection, and it was clear that that would never change.

But because of Mabel, I pay more attention to the mental health of my other chronic pain patients. I ask them about their mood and how they are handling their emotions from dealing with chronic pain. I encourage them to seek professional help when needed. I educate myself and my patients on how long-term pain puts a lot of stress on the brain, leading to depression, anxiety, and a multitude of cognitive issues including difficulty with memory or concentration.

It doesn't matter from where one's pain originates. All chronic pain patients are prone to psychological disorders, which have the potential to greatly reduce one's quality of life, not only for patients, but for their families as well. In some cases, like Mabel's, the psychological effects can surpass the chronic pain itself and become a major health disorder.

Statistics indicate that one in five adults suffering from acute and/or chronic pain, also have depression and other mood disorders. Over twenty percent of suicides are linked with ongoing pain and emotional health problems. This is why it is so important to attempt in any way to intervene when pain is overwhelming, emotions are unchecked, and lives are falling apart.

Apart from using medication, surgery, and injection to treat pain, it is essential to improve psychological wellbeing with behavioral therapy, relaxation, and coping skill training. Lifestyle changes of this type often stabilize or improve the patient's pain. Keeping positive people in one's life can also decrease suffering. It is always better for patients to have strong support from family and friends.

Dealing with chronic pain and associated anxiety and depression is a long-term battle in life. With early identification and treatment for psychological issues, proper pain management regimen, and a strong social support system, pain can be reduced to an acceptable and manageable level.

"When life is sweet, say thank you and celebrate.
When life is bitter, say thank you and grow."

A Sentinel Event

WHEN I WALKED into the procedure room one afternoon, my patient, Maureen was already lying on her stomach on the table. Earlier, I had asked my staff to check her in and get her ready so we could move the day along and catch up with our busy schedule.

Maureen was an Irish woman in her sixties. She had sandy brown long hair styled into a chignon, which isn't commonly seen nowadays on my patients. Maureen had chronic low back pain from a combination of spinal stenosis and sacroiliac joint osteoarthritis, and she routinely needed treatment for both to keep her going as well as to give her mobility to play with her grandchildren.

The sacroiliac joints have been recognized more and more as a common source for lower back pain. The sacroiliac joint typically has little motion. Small movements at the joint help with bending and shock absorption. The ligaments that circle it reinforce the network of soft tissues that surround the pelvis. Too much movement in this area causes the area to feel unstable and can lead to pain radiating to the hip and the groin while too little movement can inhibit flexibility.

Like all joints in the body, with wear and tear, the sacroiliac joint can develop arthritis and become bothersome. Steroid injections are commonly used to offer relief for patients as an alternative to conservative treatments. Maureen was scheduled to have a sacroiliac joint injection that day for that exact reason.

I walked into the treatment room and greeted her. "How are you, Maureen. Your hair looks really nice today. Did you get it colored or dyed?"

Her hair, while still in a chignon, had a different shine to it. I usually make some small talk with patients to keep their minds off the vulnerability of being on a procedure table, knowing they would soon be faced by my seemingly merciless needles.

"Aww, thank you. I didn't do anything to my hair, though. Maybe it's because I washed it this morning." Maureen laughed in her usual happy way.

"As we discussed last week during your office visit, your main discomfort now is from your sacroiliac joints. We will go ahead and treat those today.

This is different from what you had six months ago. That was an epidural steroid injection for your spinal stenosis. Has anything changed since we talked last week?"

"No."

"Great, do you have any questions before I start?"

"No."

"Okay, Maureen, let's begin with a 'TIME OUT,'" I said.

The "TIME OUT" process is part of the Universal Protocol introduced in 2003. It's performed in the procedure or operating room, immediately before the planned procedure is started. It is intended to make a last-minute check to ensure we have the correct patient, correct surgical or procedural site, and precise plan in place. It is also the time to check on the patient positioning, the need for antibiotics before the procedure, and the presence of allergies.

Studies have shown evidence that the "TIME OUT" process reduces medical errors and improves patient outcome.

In order for "TIME OUT" to really work to its fully intended effect, the process is standardized at every institution. Everyone in the procedure or operating room stops what they are doing to participate in the verification process. Ideally, the patient should be awake to participate as well.

Even though we were in a small procedure room at our own office, we still made sure we performed all the precautions and processes that we would do as if we were in a big hospital doing major surgery. Treating patients in a safe manner is always vital.

"Maureen, your full name is Maureen McCormick, correct?"

"Yes."

"Your date of birth is July 23, 1944?"

"Yes."

"Any allergies to medication, contrast, latex?"

"No."

"Are you taking any blood thinners?"

"No."

"We are doing a sacroiliac joint injection on both sides for your pain in the low back area, correct?"

"Yes, correct, doctor."

With Maureen's confirmation, I proceeded to place a needle into each of her sacroiliac joints under X-ray guidance. The procedure went smoothly, and I was satisfied with the images and my needle placement.

When I finished the procedure, I put bandages on Maureen's back.

"Maureen, take your time and be careful coming down from the procedure table. Your legs may be a little weak from lying in this position and from the numbing medicine I gave you. We can talk more when you are resting in the recovery room. My staff will assist you in moving off the procedure table now."

Maureen was very cooperative, as always, and in good spirits.

I went in my office to work on some charts as I waited for Maureen to settle down in the recovery room.

Before I even had a chance to get comfortable in my seat to record the procedure in her chart, a staff member ran into my office, pale face like a sheet of paper, as if a ghost was chasing after her.

"What's wrong?"

I knew something had gone awry.

"Dr. Shue." She closed the office door, looking dead serious.

"The patient on whom you just performed on, is not Maureen."

"What?" I jumped out of the chair, tense and afraid now.

Apparently, Maureen, the real patient, was late. Alice, my partner's patient, who was scheduled for an epidural injection for her low back, showed up at the time that Maureen was supposed to arrive. The front desk checked Alice in but did not point out this change in patients to me or the rest of the staff.

The assistant in the X-ray room, not realizing that patients had been taken out of order, took Alice into the procedure room, thinking that it was Maureen. That was when she called me in to start the procedure.

I stared at my assistant in disbelief as she was explaining the situation.

"But . . . but I saw her chignon," I murmured.

"Yes, both patients were about the same age, body structure, and had chignons."

I felt my heart racing, my head pounding and my face becoming sweaty.

"Oh no, oh no. I did the wrong procedure on the wrong patient. I am going to be sued. Oh no, I messed up big time!"

Doctors are always supposed to think about their patients first, but I couldn't help thinking about myself instead. In this day and age, every physician gets sued; It's just a matter of time. Doctors get sued often for small things, even when they are not the ones at fault. Now, I had committed a wrongdoing. I was definitely doomed. If I lost my medical license, who would take care of my patients? I was putting my patients first, if you think about it, by worrying about my own job too.

I could see a subpoena being served, and endless depositions with court appearances. I could see how I could get stressed, burned out, or fall into depression.

But how in the world could this have happened?

I was confused. No, beyond that; I was entirely flabbergasted. If I had been fooled by the chignon and the similarity of age and body types of the two patients, then why would she answer to me when I called her Maureen? We had an entire conversation about her pain. We even talked about her last office visit. I did the TIME OUT and she answered "yes" to every question, including her full name and her birthday? Wouldn't she notice that I was doing something entirely different than what she had in the past?

Maybe she was hard of hearing, or maybe she forgot what any previous injections felt like. My partner was a male doctor, for heaven's sake. Why wouldn't she think something was wrong when she was suddenly being treated by a female doctor?

By this time, my partner had been notified of what had happened. He came running in to my office urgently, expression frustrated, dark as an oncoming thunderstorm.

"What should we do? We need to figure this out," he muttered.

"Alice is happily sitting in the recovery room," my staff reported. "Should we . . . should we really tell her everything?"

If the patient thought everything went as planned, then she would never know there was a mistake. She wouldn't sue if she didn't know.

We scratched that thought right away. We decided to do the right thing and tell the truth.

"Oh, no problem." Alice listened and giggled lightheartedly as we made our desperate confession. "I feel fine. Don't worry."

That's it? I was steeling myself for a furious rant and maybe some cursing, but nothing more happened.

Alice was ready to go home, and I couldn't help but ask, "Alice, didn't you notice that it wasn't your own doctor who came into the procedure room? Why didn't you say something?"

"Oh, I thought you two were husband and wife. I thought the wife came in to help out because the husband was too busy. No matter what, I felt that you would take great care of me."

I was almost amused by her reasoning, but I was more astonished by her blind trust in us, even in the face of an unacceptable mistake on my part.

"We got lucky this time. Don't you wish all patients are as easygoing as she is?" I said to my partner as I wiped the sweat from my forehead. The dark clouds still lingered on his face.

"Well, let's hope that she has nice family members who would not talk her into changing her mind to take legal action against us," he replied warily. "She has two and a half years to think things over. That's how long someone can take legal action against doctors in New York after an event occurs."

That incident became our sentinel event. A sentinel event refers to any unanticipated event in a healthcare setting possibly resulting in serious physical or psychological injury to a patient, unrelated to the natural course of the patient's illness.

Sentinel events specifically include any events for which a recurrence would carry a risk of a serious adverse outcome. They are identified to help in root cause analysis and assist in the development of preventative measures.

The "Alice" incident prompted us to examine our "TIME OUT" process. Clearly the system had failed.

In Or Just a Waste of Time, authors Stephen Lober, MD and Sean Berry, RN pointed out that, "There are clearly intrinsic flaws in the 'TIME OUT' process as currently practiced in most hospitals today. The manner in which it is executed does not adequately account for the all-too-human foibles of distraction, complacency, and indifference. The 'TIME OUT' process should maximally engage all its participants."[27]

After the "Alice" scare, we realized that we could not trust our patients' responses. When they are on the procedure table and likely nervous, their cognitive thinking systems can potentially shut down and their hearing and other brain functions can be greatly affected. To make matters worse, some patients' blind trust in their doctor can turn them into robots, saying "yes" to every question asked.

We changed our "TIME OUT" process and had every patient actively participate to the fullest. Instead of asking them to answer yes or no, we decided to ask them to say their full names, day of birth, and what kind of procedures that they are having done and on which side of the body the procedure would be.

No "TIME OUT" process is perfect or mistake proof, but we work hard to utilize it the best we can, and faithfully go through the process before each procedure to maximize its intended benefit.

YEARS AFTER THE Alice's incident, we remained free of any other similar cases with the wrong patient, wrong side, or wrong treatment. We thanked Alice for taking us out of our comfort zone and pushing us to improve our practice. After all, our potentially destructive mistake turned into an invaluable learning experience.

Alice never changed her mind about letting me off the hook so easily. She never even mentioned the incident again. More surprisingly, she returned to the office and requested that I be her physician.

"Alice, I made a terrible mistake when I treated you last time. Why did you still trust me to taking care of you?" I asked, confused.

Alice smiled. "I don't know exactly why either, but I know that you would always treat me with honesty and compassion., Also, you liked my chignon. Isn't it a wonderful thing that I can talk about my hair when I see my doctor every time?"

27   https://www.stephenloberplasticsurgery.com/blog/2021/11/5/
timeout-or-just-a-waste-of-time-stephen-lober-md-sean-berry-rn

A Khypho What?

EVER SINCE THE chignon incident, Alice would come in from time to time to see me. We would talk about her pain and sometimes about her life. Overall, she'd been doing well with only the occasional need for an epidural injection for her low back pain.

One day, after a year without seeing her, Alice came into my office with a pained expression. By that time, she was well into her eighties. She was still a petite woman, a little more than five feet tall, yet her bright blue eyes indicated more inherent strength than her small body revealed.

"I have terrible pain in my back," she told me as she attempted to show me where the pain was, the midpoint of her spine.

I took Alice's hand and gently led her to a comfortable seat beside my desk. She walked so gingerly and slowly, with difficulty. I was stunned to see such a change in her physical state.

"Alice, tell me what happened."

"I had pneumonia about a month ago and was having lots of coughing spells and trouble breathing," she explained. "One day, while I was having a coughing fit, I felt a burst of unbearable pain in the mid-back area. The pain physically took my breath away. I thought it would get better on its own, but it never did. When I get up from bed, or even turn a little, I feel like someone is sticking a knife in my back." She showed me once more where the pain occurred. "I used to be able to take care of myself and go out with my friends from time to time, but this past month, I suddenly became an invalid. I could hardly walk to the bathroom or even cook and clean for myself.

"My friends help me with grocery shopping and stocking up my refrigerator, and all I want to do is to sit on the couch or lay in bed all day long.

"I wanted to come to see you earlier, but I had to wait for my pneumonia to get better and find myself a ride before I could come today. Please do something for me. This pain is very different from my usual problem. It's worse than anything I have experienced before."

When I put my thumb on the spine in her mid-back with slight pressure upon physical examination, Alice cried out in anguish. I jerked upright as I could imagine her suffering.

"Yes, right there. That's the right spot." It seemed to me that Alice most likely had a compression fracture of one or more vertebra in her spine, in the mid-back area.

A compression fracture refers to a collapsed vertebral body. Soft, weakened bones are at the heart of the problem. These fractures are usually caused by the bone-thinning condition, osteoporosis, especially for women over age fifty who have gone through menopause.

When bones are brittle, the vertebrae are not strong enough to support the spine, even in everyday activities. When one bends to lift an object, or miss a step, the patient can put their bones in the spine at risk of fracture. Even coughing or sneezing can cause compression fractures if one has severe osteoporosis. In this case, Alice was the recipient of the condition.

Alice is a Caucasian patient. She, along with other petite, elderly, white as well as Asian women, are at higher risk of having a compression fracture. Other risk factors include a diagnosis of osteoporosis, prominent thoracic kyphosis, which is often referred to as a hunched back, a loss of two or more inches in height, and a history of glucocorticoid therapy for diseases such as chronic asthma, rheumatoid arthritis.

In Alice's case, the severity, sudden onset, as well as the location of her issues all suggested that she had fractured a bone in her spine during that coughing spell. Patients like Alice, usually describe the discomfort as being vastly different from their usual back pain. Most of the time, an incident, such as a fall, pulling a grandchild up from the ground, or lifting heavy objects, can be identified as the root cause of the onset of a new area of pain. There are also situations where patients just don't recall an event that would result in their compromised condition.

The next step for Alice was to make the formal diagnosis and plan for treatment. An X-ray film showed the typical wedging of the fractured vertebral body.

Most compression fractures happen in the front of the vertebra. The front part of the vertebral bone usually is the part that collapses. The back of the vertebra is made of harder bone, so it stays intact. This creates a typical wedge-shaped vertebra, which can be seen on the film.

However, some fractures are far too subtle to be appreciated on the X-ray. In this case, an MRI is necessary to ascertain the whole picture. An MRI not only can pick up subtle fractures, it can also show details of how the fractures look, including if any bone fragments are pushing toward the back, creating dangerous pressure on the spinal cord. The MRI can take a good look at other structures of the spine to see if patient's pain is from other spine-related diseases.

Commonly, patients can develop both severe mid-back problems and pain shooting down the legs after an event such as a recent fall. Mid-back pain might be from a new compression fracture, while the leg problems might be from a new herniated disc in the lumbar spine. An MRI helps doctors and patients better assess the situation and allows them to develop an appropriate treatment plan and expectation for its effectiveness.

"Alice, your pain is likely to be caused by a collapsed bone in the spine. I'm sending you to have an MRI of your mid-back to make sure that is in fact the reason for your severe episode. The MRI may take a few days for the results to come back. While waiting for the results, I'll give you some medication that will help you."

She nodded. "I can't even look in the mirror anymore. I'm stooped over like the little old lady that I am." She laughed lightly. I could see that this woman hadn't given up her inner strength or sense of humor. Throughout it all, she still made me smile.

I discussed treatment options with Alice for compression fractures, which included bed rest, pain medication, and a back brace. Alice had already been homebound for the past month, so I worried about the side effects of the prolonged bed rest. Patients can sustain bone loss up to two percent a week this way. This could doubtlessly make her osteoporosis worse, which was the reason that the fracture occurred. Even worse, osteoporosis could put her at risk of more fractures in the future.

We needed to make her feel better and increase her activity level in a timely way. I encouraged her to get up from the bed and couch to walk around in the house on a regular basis. I also fitted her with a brace, which stabilized her mid and low back. The brace gives the patient support and allows them to feel less discomfort. It's worn until the fracture is mostly healed or treated with interventional procedures.

In terms of medication, the usual choices are acetaminophen, NSAIDs such as ibuprofen, naproxen, and opioids.

Patients who suffer from compression fractures are often elderly people who already have a higher risk of stomach bleeds and kidney disease. Taking NSAIDs is not the best option for most of these patients.

In Alice's case, she also has a history of atrial fibrillation, which is a condition of an irregular heartbeat. This problem can increase her chance of a clot in her heart that goes to her brain, resulting in a stroke.

To prevent a blood clot from forming, she was put on an anticoagulant, which is a blood thinner. When a patient is taking a blood thinner, she is unable to take NSAIDs because these drugs increase the tendency to bleed. For Alice, NSAIDs were not viable options.

"I have tried to take Tylenol at the maximum dosage, but it is not doing anything for my pain."

This did not surprise me. A fracture is a broken bone. I did not expect Tylenol-acetaminophen could do the trick for the severe pain related to a broken bone. I had no choice but to temporarily prescribe a low dose of opioid medication to ease her pain while she went through the process of her MRI, diagnosis, and further treatment.

I warned her about the side effects of the opioids.

"The medication can make you constipated, dizzy, drowsy, and nauseated. I worry most about the probability of a fall while on this drug. If you fall, you are likely to break other bones because your osteoporosis is already severe, and it makes your bones soft and brittle. If you hit your head, because of the blood thinner you are taking, you have a higher risk of having a bleed in the brain. Alice, you need to be extra careful while taking these pills. Please promise me you will."

She looked directly at me and firmly nodded.

I was very reluctant to put Alice on opioids, given her age and other medical problems, yet I couldn't watch her suffer either. Everything we do in medicine has pros and cons. We have to choose the lesser of the two evils, while ensuring that our patients clearly understand the risks, benefits, and precautions. This was the case with Alice who needed my care now more than ever.

When I saw Alice again, she looked ghastly as she described how unhappy she was and the degree of her pain.

"Do I have to wear this brace? It's very uncomfortable," she said as she tried to move around with it on. I had given Alice a brace long enough to support her mid and low back since her fracture was likely to be in the thoracic spine, according to my exam. This kind of brace is rigid and cumbersome and uncomfortable for most. Many patients complain about the difficulty in using them. Despite this, in this case, I felt it was necessary and had to overlook her annoyance and discomfort.

Before I could reply, Alice continued, "The opioid medication backed me up. It is terrible to have such bad constipation when I'm in severe pain already. It's just making my situation worse. I stopped taking them all together and stayed in bed all day instead."

At that point, I knew I was between the proverbial rock and a hard place. "Let's take a look at your latest MRI pictures first and see what other options we have." I wasn't surprised to hear that neither the brace nor the opioids had offered any relief to the poor lady. In this patient population, elderly women, usually in their eighties and nineties, we don't have many effective options, without specific side-effects.

On the MRI images, Alice's T12 vertebral bone looked much brighter than other bones next to it, with a wedging toward the front of the body. I showed it to Alice, noting that her T12 level compression fracture was new, and confirming it being the cause of her severe mid-backache.

"I know you can tell me now what we can do for the pain," she said. I noted that she said the word "we" as she had appointed herself a member of the treatment team. This is the best response a doctor can receive from a patient.

"Alice, I know your suffering from the compression fracture has been severe. The good news is that the fracture did not result in any nerve impingement in the spine. This means that you have the option to just give it time to heal on its own. Often it takes six weeks, but sometimes it can take about three months and even longer."

"But I'm miserable every day. It's already been a month. Tylenol has not helped. I cannot take NSAIDs or stronger pain medication. I cannot imagine how I can continue to feel like this for another two months." Alice looked at me pleadingly. "Don't you have other options for me?"

I replied, "Sometimes, patients with compression fractures can get temporary relief from a lumbar epidural steroid injection, just like what you had before for your chronic low back pain and sciatica, but the relief is usually not particularly good or long lasting. More importantly, the steroid in the injection can put you at risk of worsened osteoporosis."

Then I proceeded to tell her about another option called kyphoplasty.

"A what?" Alice asked. "Do I have to have my back cut open with this kypho—what?"

The answer for Alice was both yes and no. Her back would need a tiny four-millimeter incision but it would not be cut open. Kyphoplasty is a minimally invasive procedure. A needle the size of a spaghetti strand would be inserted through the small incision from patient's back and placed into the middle of the collapsed vertebral bone, under the constant guidance of an X-ray machine.

Through the needle, a special balloon is placed in the middle of the vertebral body. This process is done on the left and right side of the collapsed bone. Once the two balloons are in the center of the vertebral body, they are carefully inflated in small increments.

The balloon inflation has several purposes. It reduces the fracture, compacts the bone, and elevates the wedged border of the bone to restore some height of the collapsed vertebral body. It also leaves a defined cavity within the vertebral body. The balloons are then deflated and removed.

The spaces created by the balloons are then filled with PMMA, an orthopedic cement-like component used to stabilize the fracture. The cement is delivered through the two needles placed earlier, filling the deepest area first, then withdrawing the needle slightly to fill middle areas.

The pressure and amount of cement injected are closely monitored to avoid leakage into unwanted areas. When the cement hardens which usually takes only a few minutes, it provides strength and stability to the vertebra, restoring height, and relieving pain.

"Wait a minute," Alice called out as she sat straight up in her chair for the first time in weeks. "Cement in my back? Are you kidding me?"

"Don't worry, Alice. We use medical grade cement. You won't feel heavy or stiff in the area after it is placed in your vertebral bone. Most of the time, the only thing you feel is that your pain is relieved, other than some soreness from the needles.

"This procedure doesn't require a stay in the hospital. It is usually done in my office surgical suite. For sick patients with severe medical problems, it would be better to have it done at a hospital setting, with more backup support, should any complications occur.

"Kyphoplasty can be done with local anesthesia only, keeping you awake. However, I usually provide light sedation to make the experience more pleasant for patients. It helps them to know that they would remain comfortable when needles are being inserted into their bones in the spine."

Alice looked at me in awe. "You mean I can get cemented and go home when it's dry?"

"Yes. Because stitches aren't necessary, the area will just need to be bandaged, and if only one vertebra is being treated, kyphoplasty usually takes less than an hour. After your stay in the recovery room for about half an hour more, you can go home if you feel fine from the anesthesia.

"Some soreness from the needle is to be expected, which can be alleviated by placement of an ice pack. Because you may not immediately feel back to normal from the sedation anesthesia, we would like you to have someone to stay with you for the first night. The next day, you can resume your normal activities. A follow-up visit is usually scheduled for two days after the kyphoplasty, so I can remove your dressing and check on your progress."

"An incision, cement, sedation, and ice pack is a lot to think about. I would like to discuss this with my children first. Will this procedure take away all my pain?" Alice asked.

"That's the million-dollar question." I laughed and so did she. "As you know, all medical procedures can have a whole spectrum of results and responses from patients. While I don't know exactly how you will do, you have a good chance to have less pain and feel much better. The bottom line is that your fractured vertebral bone will be stronger and unlikely to collapse further."

When I first started doing kyphoplasty, it seemed to be a miracle procedure to me. I had treated a few patients with acute compression fractures, having severe back pain, and were wheelchair bound. After undergoing kyphoplasty, their pain was greatly reduced. Two of my patients had their pain almost completely disappear right after the procedure. They got up from their gurney after the sedation wore off and walked out of my office without the wheelchairs in which they arrived.

Over the years, I realized that kyphoplasty does not differ from other medical procedures in terms of the variability of patients' response. With its unquestionable effectiveness to treat a compression fracture, relief can vary from a hundred percent to a minimal degree. Most patients did report significantly reduced pain levels and had the ability to return to their normal activities.

Alice called me the next day. "I decided to have the cement operation. I think this procedure is my best choice. The other options we tried didn't work for me anyway."

I agreed with Alice. The benefits of the kyphoplasty procedure outweighed the risks for Alice, especially since she had been bed bound for far too long, and at danger of losing her existing bone density. She was even at risk of contracting infections, such as another bout of pneumonia from inactivity.

Within the week, we scheduled Alice for the procedure.

The operation took no more than forty minutes. As we followed the treatment, I explained everything to her.

When she awakened, she was in the recovery room and said, "I think you squirted the cement in the right place, because my back is already feeling better."

A smile spread across her face as she closed her eyes in relief.

About two weeks later, Alice walked into my office looking like a younger woman. Her strength had returned, her back had straightened out to some degree, and she said that she felt a twinge or two but no real pain.

"I don't know what you did, Doctor, but I feel so much better." She reached across with both arms to hug me.

"Alice, I'm so glad we could make you feel better. What I would like you to do is to see your regular physician and maybe a specialist called an endocrinologist about your osteoporosis."

I cautioned her that if her osteoporosis were not addressed, the probability of additional compression fractures would be high and although we enjoy our time together, I'd prefer that the two of us would just have a good time without worry or distress.

According to the International Osteoporosis Foundation, one in three women and one in eight men are prone to osteoporosis by age fifty. The US National Osteoporosis Foundation reports that over 44 million Americans are likely to develop osteoporotic conditions as they grow older. There are more than two million fractures related to osteopenia or osteoporosis annually in the United States, including hips, forearms, vertebral bodies, and other sites in the body. That means that more men and women are likely to have osteoporotic fractures than heart disease, stroke, or breast cancer.

Osteoporosis is a common problem that causes bones to become abnormally thin, weakened, and easily fractured. Women are at a higher risk for osteoporosis after menopause due to lower levels of estrogen, a female hormone that helps to maintain bone mass. Fortunately, preventive treatments are available that can help to maintain or increase bone density.

A few factors are important in the prevention of osteoporosis.

An adequate intake of calcium, and vitamin D, is essential in helping to maintain proper bone formation and density. Experts often recommend that men over seventy years and postmenopausal women consume 800 international units of vitamin D each day. This dose appears to reduce bone loss and fracture rate in older women and men who have adequate calcium intake. Although the optimal intake has not been clearly established in premenopausal women or in younger men with osteoporosis, 600 international units of vitamin D daily is generally suggested.

Drinking alcohol more than two drinks a day can increase the risk of fracture due to an increased risk of falls and poor nutrition. Restricting caffeine or salt has not been proven to prevent bone loss in people who consume an adequate amount of calcium.

Smoking cigarettes is known to accelerate bone loss. One study suggested that women who smoke one pack per day throughout adulthood have a five to ten percent reduction in bone density by menopause, resulting in an increased risk of fracture.

Exercise may decrease fracture risk by improving bone mass in premenopausal women and helping to maintain bone density for women after menopause. Most experts recommend exercising for at least thirty minutes a day, by taking a brisk walk, three times a week.

The benefits of exercise are quickly lost when a person stops their routine. A regular, weight bearing exercise regimen that a person enjoys improves the chances that the person will continue it over the long term.

When people think about hip fracture, many recognize it as the beginning of the end for many elderly patients. Data published in Osteoporosis International in 2000 revealed that while hip fracture puts a patient at about sevenfold risk of dying in about four years, a vertebral fracture puts a patient at higher risk of about ninefold of death in the same length of time. After first vertebral body fracture, the likelihood of having another vertebral fracture goes up fivefold. After two fractures, it rises to 12-fold. After three or more, it increases to 75-fold.[28]

With multiple compression fractures, the body begins to show the effects. The strength and shape of the spine can change. One loses height because the spine is shorter. Most compression fractures happen in the front of the vertebra, creating a typical wedge-shaped vertebra. This can lead to the stooped posture known colloquially as a dowager's hump. Its medical term is kyphosis.

28   https://link.springer.com/journal/198/volumes-and-issues

This curvature is not only a matter of appearance, but it can also affect a person's ability to breathe. A single level thoracic vertebral compression fracture in the mid back can cause nine percent loss of lung capacity. The degree of kyphosis is significantly related to risk of death related to lung function.

As people live longer, osteoporosis and related fractures have become a major health issue. For woman over the age of eighty, about 80 percent have osteoporosis and 40 percent of them have sustained at least one level of vertebral compression fracture.

The most important thing to do for a patient with known osteoporosis is to have an awareness of the risk for fractures to facilitate early diagnosis, including vertebral compression fracture.

Not every patient needs intervention for vertebral compression fracture. In fact, I have seen patients came to me for other spine-related problems. Their MRI films would show compression fractures that were already healed. Most of them could not even recall any painful episodes correlating to the fractures.

Some other patients would present themselves with new fractures but minimal discomfort. They were able to go about their daily business without difficulty. Some of them had to take medication which were highly effective and did not give them any major side effects. For these patients, kyphoplasty is not indicated. Their fractures would heal on their own, while their lives were minimally affected.

One of my kyphoplasty patients recently asked, "Since the other bones in my spine are also very soft and weak and may break in the future anyway, can't you just put cement in all of them to prevent the fracture from happening?"

"That would not be a good idea," I had to admit. "Kyphoplasty is only indicated for painful, acute, or subacute compression fractures. This means that if the fracture is too old, usually more than six months, it is already healed. Kyphoplasty is not indicated because it can no longer raise the collapsed bone. Chances are that a healed fracture does not cause any pain."

If a patient still experiences backache with the history of an old compression fracture, other sources of pain need to be considered and investigated. On the other hand, as I told my patient, kyphoplasty is not done for prophylactic purposes, such as to prevent bone from collapsing in the future, even if osteoporosis is severe and fracture is likely.

Whether a new and unpleasant vertebral compression fracture should be treated by kyphoplasty, or when to offer this option to patient, still sparks disagreement within the medical community.

Doctors who prefer conservative treatments argue: Why put a patient who is usually frail, elderly, with multiple medical problems, through an invasive procedure when the fracture would heal on its own? There are studies showing that once a vertebral body is cemented, the levels above and below are at higher risks of fracture.

On the other side of the debate, doctors argue that the healing process can take up to three months, or even longer. If pain from the vertebral fracture is severe and uncontrolled, it can make patients bedbound or housebound. This can be a risk factor for a variety of medical problems, such as infection, bone loss, anxiety, depression, diminished self-esteem, further dependency on others, and general health deterioration. These medical problems can become fatal, especially in this particularly vulnerable patient group. Once a patient has a fracture, the chance of having another fracture increases regardless of any kind of treatment choices.

A study published in the Journal of Bone and Joint Surgery in 2013, by Dr. Andrew Chen, analyzed data on more than 72,000 patients with vertebral compression fractures. The study compared how patients do if they underwent kyphoplasty vs. no procedural treatment. The estimated three-year survival rates were 42 percent for nonoperative treatment and 60 percent for the kyphoplasty groups, respectively.[29]

Results also concluded that patients in the kyphoplasty group had the shortest hospital stay and the highest hospital charges (cost of kyphoplasty itself is high because of equipment and operating room use) but were the least likely to have had pneumonia and decubitus ulcers.

I once had a patient in her late eighties who sustained a vertebral compression fracture, seven months before she came to see me. She was sent to me to wean off her opioids. By the time I saw her, the pain in her back from the fracture had mostly resolved. However, she looked confused, unable to communicate verbally, with obvious cognitive impairments.

The family members and her son, who accompanied her to the visit told me, "She used to be an active person, able to carry a normal conversation. After she had the fracture, she was put on opioids for her pain. She was never the same. She seemed to have lost her identity. We would like her opioids to be weaned off and she can return to us as herself again."

With the help of the family, the patient successfully tapered down and eventually stopped taking the opioids. According to her son, she improved cognitively, but never returned to her original state before the fracture and her prolonged period of opioids use. They wished that they had been given the possibility of kyphoplasty as a treatment option at the early stage of the process.

There was no way for anyone to know what exactly had caused this patient's cognitive decline. We all wondered if she had kyphoplasty done

29   https://www.jbjs.org/reader.php?rsuite_id=1195309&native=1&source=The_Journal_of_Bone_and_Joint_Surgery/95/19/1729/abstract&topics=sp#info

to improve her pain and avoided the seven months of opioid use, would the outcome be different? We will never know. But I believe it is essential to educate and provide patients with kyphoplasty as a treatment option and help them decide if this is the best choice for them.

"I know you won't believe me, but the highest form of Human Excellence is to question oneself and others." — Socrates

The Pharma Reps Appear

WE CAN BE managing a very full day of work when a pharmaceutical representative from any number of pharmaceutical companies appear with samples of a new product.

They are well-dressed, good-looking men and women, poised and ready to explain anything I want to know about the new drug they would want me to consider for use in my practice. They represent the company they work for as they are the well-trained face of the pharmaceutical community.

In an ideal world, as physicians, we would keep up with the newest drug developments by reading academic journal articles and attending scientific symposiums. We would have weekly medical conferences to discuss patient management cases with colleagues and learn from each other's success and failures. That was how I kept myself up to date during my residency and fellowship.

After I left the Ivory Tower of the academic world, and went into private practice, I was on my own. I am not sure how other doctors in private practice handle it. For me, the daily grind of seeing patients, managing the business, paying bills, and juggling with personal and family needs have taken over my life.

Read a journal article? That's probably the most effective method to put me to sleep if I accumulate enough guilt and finally pick up a professional magazine. Pharmaceutical reps come along and fill the void.

In a JAMA editorial in 2017, the author pointed out: "There are potential advantages to pharmaceutical detailing, which refers to pharmaceutical reps visiting doctors' office. Although physicians can find prescribing information using online resources, one report estimated that it takes nearly ten years for evidence from reviews, research articles, and textbooks to be widely adopted by the medical community. Pharmaceutical companies have the resources, national workforce, and financial incentive to address this issue. Detailing may accelerate adoption of novel therapies."[30]

Nowadays, all promotional materials provided by any pharmaceutical company must be approved by the FDA and the company's legal and compliance department. Reps are also well aware of the fact that they cannot make false claims in order to promote their products. Any indications or disease states other than what is approved by the FDA cannot be mentioned in the presentation. If the product is not a controlled substance, samples are frequently offered.

In short, the reps provide condensed and precise information on a particular drug or medical product in a quick and easy format for doctors, but the doctors are almost always too busy to talk to the reps.

No problem. A doctor has to eat lunch, correct? Let's meet when the doctor eats. Lunch will be provided by the drug company as a token of appreciation for the doctor's time. Isn't that a solution where everyone benefits?

I have been fully aware of the different types of information offered by peer review journal articles versus information presented by commercial companies. In order for a new medication to be put on the market, it has to go through three phrases of clinical trials. The clinical trial data can be presented in various ways, depending on what needs to be emphasized.

One time, one pharmaceutical rep presented me with two bar graphs with a drastic difference in heights of the two bars, giving readers a sense that one product was far superior to the other. As I closely examined the graph, the numerical difference was a mere three percent, which was less significant than what the contrast the bar graph tried to convey.

On another occasion, I also saw how a study result showed great data, yet we realized in the fine print that only twenty patients were involved in the study. It is usually difficult to argue such a small sample size that can yield clinically significant results.

I do not point out these little tricks that I figure out on the promotional materials to the company reps. After all, they do not do the clinical trials or analyze the data. They do not design the pamphlets. They probably are taught exactly what to say or what not to say to doctors regarding their products. They are simply hard-working people doing their job. Why make their day more difficult than it already is? Ultimately, I have the freedom to prescribe the drug, or not. I still make my own decision as a physician. I like to believe that with my own critical thinking capabilities, I can take away the knowledge I need and leave the influence of the commercial companies behind.

We see reps come and go. Sometimes they come by the office just to tell us about changes and to drop off samples. Most of the salespeople are friendly, mild mannered, and never pushy. I would spend a few minutes with them. Give them a signature in exchange for medication samples. Simple and straightforward business.

That, however, was not the case with Brian.

Brian came to us from one of the largest pharmaceutical companies in the country. For his first visit, he scheduled a lunch with my staff and arrived with a good spread of food in our lunchroom. I usually would not schedule lunch break for myself. I would spend about five minutes gulping down my food and keep seeing patients. I like to get work done and go back home to my family at the end of the day, as early as possible.

On that day, I swiftly got my plate of food and was ready to hear Brian's pitch for his company's newest and greatest product.

"Why don't you enjoy your lunch? I am the kind of rep who puts a doctor's health and wellbeing ahead of my job. Please eat first. I will just give you a noticeably short talk about my product afterwards. It won't take up much of your time at all. I promise."

Brian sat across the table from me, smiling. Wow, what a considerate fellow. I appreciated it. He kept his promise and watched me clear my plate in three minutes before he educated me about his product with great enthusiasm. He even offered a power point presentation. The demonstration showed how the new product compared to other brands and existing generic medicines, detailing several recent study results.

Brian then moved on to tell us how a patient could get insurance coverage for the medication, and what the co-pays would be with the company coupon and discount program. He told us how he and his company could help our patients get prior authorization, which is the hurdle for insurance companies to agree to pay for these often-expensive new drugs.

Before the authorization would kick in, Brian would provide medication samples to distribute to those who choose to try this drug. That way, the patient would not have to wait to get the therapy. If the patient had side effects, he or she could stop the medication and avoid having to spend any money, up front, for a month's supply of medication.

All the information was reasonable and important. However, Brian seemed to have forgotten the second part of his promise, which was to keep the talk short and sweet. My patients were filling up the waiting area and I was itching to go to them.

Well, there is no free lunch, remember? I looked at the smoothie that came with the lunch, gulped it down, feeling the satisfied happiness of my stomach.

Just let him do his job, I thought. My time is the price I paid for this lunch.

Brian concluded his conversation with us by saying that his product was completely new and there was no generics available. Drug companies spend a fortune to develop a new drug. They need to make their money back, for the new drug, and the many drugs that consumed millions of dollars in development but never made it to the market. Pharmaceutical companies often bear the bad reputation as money thirst monsters.

However, it is a straightforward and reasonable concept. If there is no profit, there will be no incentives for new drug development. That would be bad news for everyone, especially for patients.

Pharmaceutical companies can make lots more money when they can mark up the price before their drug patent expires. That's why the quick sale is so important. In order to capitalize on the new drug in town, they must sell the product within a period of time before generics come in at a considerably smaller cost.

We wrapped it up in every way—food, drink, and conversation. Brian left us with a stack of pharma magazines, pamphlets, and the like, with a promise to come back soon again.

He came back, too much and too soon. For a while, Brian would come back every week. He made sure that he had face time with me during each visit.

"Dr. Shue, tell me. What is your experience with the product in the past week?"

Brian turned out to be a close talker. He leaned over my face. His eyeballs were right next to mine. I could see each fine blood vessel weaving through them.

I stepped back a little each time I met with him.

"Humm, I have not had a chance to use it in the past week."

That obviously was not a good answer.

"Can you think of a few patients in the past week for whom you could have used the product? In what situation would you think of using our product? Do you use our competitors' products? Please remember the great data that our product had shown in recent studies. Just to remind you a little bit."

In one quick motion, he proceeded to pull out his computer tablet and present his PowerPoint, yet again.

I understood those were all good questions. However, when they were asked repeatedly, every week, I could not help but feel that I was being interrogated, and that was not a "feel good" experience.

If my waiting room was jam packed, it did not matter. Brian would quietly wait in the waiting room. One hour? A piece of cake. Two hours? No problem. He would wait until the crowd cleared.

One time, I was completely immersed in my work and forgot that a staff member had told me that Brian was waiting for me. When I finished everything at six p.m., ready to leave the office, he was still there waiting. I had no reason not to give him a few minutes. Who could say no to such a dedicated worker?

"Please tell me, doctor. What is your experience with the product in the past week?"

Not again. But Brian asked me this question again and again, without fail. I knew there was nothing wrong for me to tell him. "No, I have not used any of your product. I don't have time for this. Please do not come to this office again."

But obviously, my skin was not thick enough. How could I use his enthusiasm and love of his job to go against him? I just wish I had somewhere to hide. Furthermore, I realized that I did feel the slightest guilt because I did not use his product.

Guilt would be total nonsense. I was annoyed with myself for feeling like I should have listened more to Brian. But I was doing the right thing for my patients, and for society, by choosing the best medication for my patients based on my own medical knowledge and keeping the price tag in mind.

When I was a medical student, I was taught that we needed to have a social responsibility to watch how much money we ask our patients and the health care system to spend. My professor in internal medicine who trained me while I was in medical school, had ingrained this doctrine in my head. I was taught to order labs and studies only when needed, and always use generic medication unless there is a clear advantage of using a brand name one.

We, as doctors, need to be the conscience and influence on society. When the total medical cost is lower, it is less of a financial burden on everyone. When the escalating cost puts too much stress on the society, guess what would happen? The cost will be cut. And that would affect everyone, patients, and doctors. We are all on the same boat.

As Dr. Nicole Van Groningen pointed out in her article that appeared in the Washington Post on June 13, 2017:[31]

"On a national scale, the financial burden imposed by branded drugs is enormous. Current estimates place our prescription drug spending annually, and branded drugs are almost entirely to blame: Though they constitute only 10 percent of prescriptions, they account for 72 percent of total drug spending. Even modest reductions in our use of branded prescription drugs could translate to billions of dollars in national health-care savings."

To lower the cost of health care by using generics is important, but things are always more complicated than we like. Herein lies the problem. There is an ongoing war between brand and generic medication. Some pharmaceutical companies claim that their brand name products are still far better than generic drugs while generic drug companies insist their products provide the same care at less cost.

31   https://www.washingtonpost.com/opinions/big-pharma-gives-your-doctor-gifts-then-your-doctor-gives-you-big-pharmas-drugs/2017/06/13/5bc0b550-5045-11e7-b064-828ba60fbb98_story.html

A February 2018 article in Fortune Magazine reported: "Generic drugs diverge from the originals far more than most of us believe. For starters, it's not as if the maker of the original pharmaceutical hands over its manufacturing blueprint when its patent runs out or is challenged. The patent reveals the components, but it doesn't explain how to make the drug. In reality, manufacturing a generic requires reverse engineering, and the result is an approximation rather than a duplicate of the original."[32]

The FDA's rules effectively acknowledge that the agency's definition of bio equivalence is surprisingly broad: A generic's maximum concentration of active ingredient in the blood must not fall more than 20 percent below or 25 percent above that of the brand name. This means a potential range of 45 percent, by that measure, among generics labeled as being the same.

There are other differences. The generic must contain the same active ingredient as the original. But the additional ingredients, known as excipients, can be different and are often of lower quality. Those differences can affect what's called bio availability—the amount of drug that could potentially be absorbed into the bloodstream.

As the American Heart Association noted in 2017, "Some additives traditionally thought to be inert, such as alcohol sugars, cyclodextrans and polysorbate-80, may alter a drug's dissolution, thereby impacting its bio availability."

In the world of medicine, the effectiveness of a drug is the bottom line. Some brand name drugs do not have a generic equivalent because the patents are still in place. Some do seem more effective than the generic versions.

When I prescribe brand name medication for patients because other generic alternatives have failed to produce results, it is often met with resistance from insurance companies.

The drug reps are happy, but the insurance companies are not because they naturally do not want to pay for the extra cost associated with the brand name products. To discourage the use of brand name drugs, a process called prior authorization is required.

Patients have to have tried and failed with a few other medications before they are allowed to get the brand name medication. In addition, they must have a certain specific medical diagnosis to be eligible. Doctors have to fill out form after form to prove that the patient has, in fact, fit all of the above criteria. To make things worse, each insurance company has its own paperwork and requirements, making this process time consuming and confusing.

When patients do not get their medication on time, they lay blame on the doctors for causing the delay and the failure of authorization. And do you know what? The patients are correct.

32   https://fortune.com/2018/02/15/warren-buffett-teva-berkshire-hathaway/

After seeing patients all day, I am not always able to go through every piece of paperwork and fill it out properly on time. I wish I could do better. I understand where the insurance companies are coming from, but I wish the process were easier and doctors would have more say in which medication their patients should take, instead of being determined by a check list, created by the insurance companies.

The pharmaceutical company representatives also come in to help in this situation. The co-pay coupon cards can decrease the monthly cost, sometimes down to zero. The prior authorization department can help with the paperwork. The company has contracts with specialty pharmacies which can further facilitate the process.

Are all of the above, along with the occasional lunch worth the trouble of dealing with drug reps? Every time I saw Brian in the office, I wondered.

One day, when the lunch order was brought in for our drug rep meeting, a patient saw it all and exclaimed, "Oh, my Lord, is that how you eat every day?" I was not sure what she had imagined when she only saw a couple of brown bags.

The lunches are usually capped at approximately twenty dollars per person. The drug rep must document the cost and have everyone who attends the meeting sign a special form. The total dollar amount spent on each physician is available as public information. This is known as the "Sunshine Act" reporting.

The Sunshine Act, passed in 2010, requires most makers of drugs and medical supplies to report all payments, gifts, and other services worth ten dollars or more that they provide to health professionals.

Nearly 95 percent of U.S. physicians accept gifts, meals, payments, travel, and other services from companies that make the drugs and medical products they prescribe, according to the New England Journal of Medicine. This had been a common practice for decades, and studies show it affects doctors' prescribing decisions.[33]

The Sunshine Act is aimed to discourage pharmaceutical companies' interaction and influence on physician prescribing habit.

I searched myself on the Sunshine Act, just out of curiosity. There was a dollar amount next to my name. The amount was much bigger than I expected. But the days of trips and vacations at the hand of the pharma companies are long over. Even complimentary pen and paper pads are banned. How did the companies spend all the money on me by just bringing in lunch?

I wasn't satisfied with the lack of explanation of the website regarding how the money was spent on each physician. A layman can easily assume that

---

33   https://www.denverpost.com/2014/07/11/sunshine-act-will-reveal-drug-companies-giving-gifts-to-your-doctor/

it was given as cash to the doctor when the truth was that my pocket did not get any fatter by one single cent. I never saw any gifts materialize other than medication samples and brochures for the patients.

I did not like to imagine what my patients would think when they saw the data on this website. To make my life easier, I asked my staff members to reduce sponsored lunches to the minimum. That's how they win. I marveled at how the Sunshine Act has achieved its purpose, at least, in my case.

I still allow pharmaceutical representatives to come to my office and drop off educational material. Studies show it definitely affects doctors' prescribing decisions. I knew that, but I am extra cautious and critical of the information provided. I knew it was untrue when a rep tried to tell me there was no generic equivalent to his product. I rolled my eyes when a rep advised me to increase the opioid dosage above the conversion calculation to achieve better results and make a patient happier. When a company tried to talk me into their lucrative speaker program, I did not take the bait because I disagreed with how that medication was being promoted. Even with somebody as aggressive as Brian, I did not give in to prescribing medication that I deemed inappropriate for my patients. I was confident in my ability to handle it myself.

ONE DAY, I came across the article in the New Yorker by Patrick Keefe, named "The Family That Built an Empire of Pain." The entire article was a fascinating read. What caught my eyes was the part where Keefe described: Doctors who prescribed OxyContin were beginning to report that patients were coming to them with symptoms of withdrawal (itching, nausea, the shakes) and asking for more medication. *David Haddox*, Purdue Pharma's former vice president of health policy, had an answer. In a 1989 paper, Haddox coined the term "pseudo-addiction."[34]

As a management pamphlet distributed by Purdue explained, pseudo-addition "seems similar to addiction, but is due to unrelieved pain." The pamphlet continues, "Misunderstanding of this phenomenon may lead the clinician to inappropriately stigmatize the patient with the label 'addict.'"

"Pseudo-addiction." I remember while I was in training in the 2000s, how this term was discussed among professors, colleagues, during patient cases. I made a mental note to remind myself not to let these poor patients suffer by mistaking them as addicts.

More than ten years later, I found out this was just part of the scheme for a pharmaceutical company to encourage doctors to give more OxyContin to the masses.

34   https://www.newyorker.com/magazine/2017/10/30/the-family-that-built-an-empire-of-pain

I was aghast. I didn't think I was immune to the influence of pharmaceutical companies' tactics. But I did not realize how ignorant I was about their influence on one doctor—me!

How should I re-evaluate and determine my physician-pharmaceutical company relationship? Like any relationship, there isn't a straightforward simple answer. Also, like any relationship, nothing should be taken for granted. I have to keep an alert mind and critical view.

"Physician, heal thyself thus you help your patient too. Let his best
help be with his own eyes, the man who makes himself well."
— Friedrich Nietzsche c. 1884

ALL IN A DAY'S WORK

ON AN EARLY fall day, I began my first day of work as an anesthesiologist
for a gastroenterology specialist, Dr. Roth. His office was about forty miles
from where I lived. It would take me more than an hour in the morning to
commute there and even longer to drive back home after work because of
rush hour traffic. I didn't like driving long distances, but in this case, I didn't
mind too much because I still had to pay my bills.

I had just started a pain management office with my partner. The practice
was still too young to take care of itself and I needed outside income to dump
into the "black hole" for it to survive.

Since my office patient load was still light, I decided to work every day
in the morning from seven-thirty a.m. to early afternoon for a full shift of
anesthesia work. Then I would go back to my own office and see patients
from three p.m. to around seven p.m.

Dr. Roth did procedures in his own surgical suite. My job was to evaluate
the patients for sedation and then, to keep them sleeping comfortably and
safely while Dr. Roth performed a colonoscopy or endoscopy. These processes
are usually referred to as office-based procedures and sedation.

I arrived extra early to get well situated to ensure my first day would go
smoothly. I set up the anesthesia station to my satisfaction.

Our first patient arrived on time. I introduced myself and got the
intravenous line started. The patient was ready to go in the procedure suite.
Everything went very smoothly; I was cruising along. A perfect morning, or
so I thought. Suddenly, I heard some commotion outside of the procedure
suite.

It seemed that a couple of people were talking loudly to each other. Then I
noticed Tina, the office manager, coming by and she quickly closed the door
of the procedure room.

The noise outside grew louder, sprinkled by some faint yelling and even
cursing. Then something metallic hit the floor. Or was it glass?

Before I could think about what was going on, the door swung open.
Dr. Roth strode in, looking apologetic. He said to both the patient and me,
"Sorry about the delay. We can start now."

After the patient was sedated and sound asleep, which meant it was now safe for us to talk, Dr. Roth looked at me and said, "I'm sure you heard the noise out there. It was just a patient making a scene for no reason."

Oh, that was what it was. I gave him a sympathetic look. I knew exactly how it was to have unreasonable patients in the office. I bet everybody in the business of health care can recount a couple of jaw dropping stories about difficult patients. I also had my own collection of stories, and I was excited to take some time to trade stories. I searched the room, hoping to meet the eyes of the nurse or Dr. Roth in order to gather some more clues and get them talking. Yet, both remained quiet.

After the procedure was complete, there was an awkward pause. Dr. Roth looked at me taking a deep breath. "Well," he said in a solemn voice, "that was my previous anesthesiologist."

Hmm; something didn't sound right.

Did he mean what just happened outside had something to do with me? Did I take that person's job? The person who was very angry, and just made a scene out there?

I thought that I was just an audience, getting ready to enjoy a nice show on the stage. All of a sudden, the music cut, and the spotlight shined upon me. I was caught with popcorn in my mouth, completely unprepared to be part of the performing cast. This was only my first day working here. I wasn't supposed to be involved in any drama yet!

Patients kept coming and procedures kept going, but now things were awkwardly silent. I stayed calm and professional, and focused on my job. Yet, inside my head were a thousand bees buzzing around with only questions, no answers.

Who was the bad guy in this case? Everyone knows that employees come and go, but how did this one end with such drama and bad blood? Was I getting myself in trouble working here? Maybe I had taken away somebody's job. Would that person be waiting for me outside to attack me as I left the office? I felt a little paranoid, but the whole situation (and my imagination) made it seem like a scene from a movie.

The rest of the day went smoothly, unremarkable and boring. I've learned to appreciate a boring workday. It means everything has gone very well. To my relief, nobody ran toward me to yell at me, or even look at me as I left the office and walked to my car in the parking lot.

Because I managed to keep his days peaceful enough, Dr. Roth decided that I was a good anesthesiologist to keep. As I got to know everyone in the office, I wondered if I would learn little bits about my predecessor, but somehow, the person and the event just faded away.

One summer day, ten years later, I happened to work with Dr. Roth again. By this time, he was a partner of a well-run ambulatory surgical center.

With Dr. Roth's recommendation to his other partners, I had taken the job to ensure sufficient anesthesia staffing for the center. We would only work together from time to time. On this day, we exchanged pleasantries, asked about each other's families, and went on to marvel how ten years had gone by since we first worked together.

I looked at Dr. Roth and smiled. "You know, my memory is going downhill, but I remember very well about the first day I worked with you."

His eyes opened wide. Then, he chuckled and said, "Yes, me too. And you were very cool about it that day." Tina, the office manager at Dr. Roth's office, was also working at the center. We gathered Tina and the two of them recounted the story to me.

The subject was Dr. Hernandez. The woman in question was originally from Cuba and was a doctor there. She came to the US on a boat with little in her pocket. Newly arrived in the US, she had to start off doing odd jobs—any job that she could find. How she overcome her financial difficulties, the impossible hardship to pass the multitude of examinations, to apply to medical residency programs while having to make ends meet, nobody knew the details. She had managed to work at Dr. Roth's office for a few years, was well liked, providing safe and good care to patients.

However, things started to change a few months before I started working there. She got involved in an affair with a married man. When the relationship grew sour, she became emotionally unstable, and started showing signs that made the office staff worry if she was still capable of providing safe care to patients on the job.

Dr. Roth voiced his concern with her but saw no improvement. After more discussions, she agreed that she would leave, but would stay for another couple weeks in order for Dr. Roth to find a new anesthesiologist. When the doctor found me, and decided on my start date, he emailed her, but she did not reply. He also called her, but nobody answered the phone. Finally, Dr. Roth left messages on voice mail on her phone and informed her that she did not have to come to work any longer, giving her a specific date as the end of her service.

That specific date was my first day of work at Dr. Roth's office. As I was getting things ready with the patient in the procedure room, Dr. Hernandez walked in the office as usual, holding a cup of coffee. As she walked through the office, toward the procedure suite, Tina spotted her. Tina, who came from a background of military training, immediately realized that action and damage control were warranted.

Tina wasted no time. She ran to notify Dr. Roth, then lunged at the door of the procedure suite to snap it shut. Dr. Roth sprinted out of his office and got between Dr. Hernandez and the procedure room just in time. He explained to her how he found another anesthesiologist and how he tried multiple ways to inform her about the change. This explanation only angered Dr. Hernandez who apparently was unprepared for her sudden loss of employment.

In a rage, she threw her fresh hot cup of coffee at Dr. Roth. She was then pulled away by other staff members when she continued to curse and act aggressively toward him and the others. The rage, crying, screaming, and the commotion went on as she entered the parking lot, and the police had to be called to handle the problem.

"The police thought that she was Dr. Roth's mistress and we had to do a lot of explaining." Tina laughed. "What a huge mess."

"Two years after she left my office," Dr. Roth said, "I had a conversation with a colleague of mine. He said his anesthesiologist literally broke down at work. She shut herself in a room and cried for eight hours straight in his office. The doctor had to cancel all patient procedures for the day because there was no anesthesia service. Guess what? It was Dr. Hernandez."

To this day, I think of Dr. Hernandez. Not because of the drama she created; I just felt sorry for her, as a colleague and fellow physician.

In the United States, a medical doctor's license invariably means years of rigorous academic requirement and demanding clinical training. Dr. Hernandez, like the rest of us, had earned her medical degree and license with plenty of blood, sweat, and probable tears, if not more. However, all of it was put in jeopardy when she was unable to balance work and personal life. She already lost two stable jobs that we know of. Worse yet, she could have potentially done harm to patients and subsequently lose her license to practice medicine altogether.

Work and personal life balance is important for everyone. However, it has a great deal of impact on health care professionals. We take care of people at our work. Our own lack of wellbeing can lead to lack of judgment, resulting in others' pain, suffering, inconvenience, complications, or even death.

One time, I slammed my index finger in my car door. The pain was sudden and excruciating. In order to distract myself, I ran around the parking lot to take my mind of my pain. A friend who happened to be there, looked at my finger with a mashed nail hanging on a thread, full of blood and said, "Calm down. You are a pain doctor, for heaven's sake. Are you that upset over something like this?"

I was not sure which one was more hurtful, the searing pain in my mangled finger, or the comment, made by an adult with a Ph.D. degree.

Who says doctors don't feel the same way that everyone else does?

I really hurt! The awful experience happened to affect my patients too, because I could only use my left hand to do procedures for a few days. My injured finger was too swollen to fit into sterile gloves.

I never saw any doctor for treatment of my injured hand. I was too busy with my work and other responsibilities. It was much later that, by chance, I found out that I had actually fractured the finger when it got slammed in the car door.

Like everyone else, doctors have personal problems. We get sick, divorced, have custody battles, infidelity, disabled children, deaths in our families. Yet, working sixty to ninety or even more hours per week, immersed in our patients' pain means we often have no time to deal with our own. I'm always surprised by how often non-medical people tell me they are shocked that doctors have the same mental health issues and personal problems as everyone else.

Many people in or out of the medical profession believe the public doesn't need to know that doctors are in distress, as if a healer being in pain is shameful and would frighten patients. A large number of them are seriously uncomfortable with the subject.

When patients have appointments with their doctors, they are often in pain or some degree of discomfort. The last thing they want to face is a doctor who displays anything but perfect professional behavior.

Doctors are expected to smile, be kind and compassionate. No matter what is going on in their personal lives, it must be left outside of the consultation or operating room. Even if a doctor encounters a difficult patient and is physically and emotionally drained, he or she has to pretend that nothing has happened when the doctor sees the next patient.

Remember Mabel, Aaron, and Bertha?

As our days are overfilled with clinical care responsibility, paperwork, deadlines, fear of lawsuits, and the like, we forget to take care of ourselves, physically, emotionally, and mentally. With time, this type of emotional pain can result in physician burnout.

Burned-out physicians can be harmful to their patients and to themselves. Many physicians appear to function fairly well or think they are doing well. "Those suffering from burnout or depression often have grave delusional thinking," Mick Oreskovich, MD, a Seattle psychiatrist, said. "They are going to work thinking that they're still doing a good job. They are often the last person in the room to know how depressed they are."[35]

While struggling with burnout, doctors usually communicate less effectively with patients, which is a major concern. After all, medicine is about listening to patients and connecting with them, in addition to providing good treatment plans.

These doctors may make little effort to listen to their patients. Consequently, they can be impatient and irritable when dealing with patient issues. This leads to lower patient satisfaction, improper treatment, and poor patient care outcome.

35   https://www.medscape.com/viewarticle/887467

A study done at the Mayo Clinic, sponsored by the American Medical Association found that patients of exhausted physicians had significantly lower patient satisfaction scores.

Patients are less cooperative to doctors whom they do not like, which can further reduce treatment compliance and the quality of care that patients receive.

It has been shown that patients are more likely to sue physicians whom they think are not taking good care of them. In a review of closed claims from 2015 to 2018, by The Doctors Company, a medical malpractice insurer owned by physicians, poor communication between doctor and patient was noted as a risk management issue in almost forty percent of the cases.[36]

According to a 2018 analysis, also performed by the AMA, burned-out physicians have been linked to more medical errors and higher malpractice risks, as well as sub-optimal care.[37]

Poor patient review and lawsuits exacerbate physician's stress and escalate this vicious cycle of burnout.

Burned-out physicians not only do harm to their patients, but also put themselves in harm's way.

The impact of burnout on physicians' personal lives has been linked to a higher rate of car accidents, poor health, and weight gain. Relationships with family and friends tend to suffer. Physicians' marriages can be significantly harmed by burnout. A 2017 study linked work and home conflict with burnout in both male and female physicians.

Burnout is a profoundly serious mental health problem. Like other mental health issues, if we ignore it, it generally gets worse. It can lead to depression and self-destructive behavior, including violent outbursts, alcoholism, drug addiction, and suicide.

In the article named "Fighting a Silent Epidemic" published on the website healthtrustpg.com, it quotes that, "A 2015 Mayo Clinic study revealed that more than 7 percent of nearly 7,000 doctors had considered taking their own lives in the past 12 months, compared with 4 percent of professionals in other fields. Approximately 400 doctors a year commit suicide." A staggering number of Americans lose their doctors to suicide each year. Many doctors, myself included, have lost a colleague to suicide.[38]

The author of this article also points out that, "physicians agree that . . . much of their stress is rooted in the changing healthcare landscape. Not only must they struggle with serving an aging patient population with higher

36   https://www.thedoctors.com/articles/hospitalist-closed-claims-study/
37   https://jamanetwork.com/journals/jamainternalmedicine/
fullarticle/2698144
38   https://healthtrustpg.com/?s=Fighting+a+Silent+Epidemic&post_
type=page%2Cpost&cat=&order=desc

rates of chronic disease, but they are also pressed to provide better, more efficient care to patients at lower costs and with fewer resources. Some of the biggest sources of frustration for physicians are the cumbersome electronic health records (EHRs) . . . pre-approval requirements from health insurers for services, as well as quality metrics built into the Affordable Care Act."

Burn out can inconspicuously slip in my daily routine. As much as I love my profession, I would have moments of wanting to give up medicine altogether, only to recognize that I need to step back and take a break from the daily grind. Yet, I cannot run away from any of the problems. For me, the deepest discontent comes from regulatory mandates and insurance pre-approval requirements. It severely interferes with physicians' autonomy, increases the burden of clerical work and overhead cost for doctors and their staff, and decreases patient satisfaction.

For example, The Centers for Medicare & Medicaid Services published its new rules regarding lumbar epidural steroid injection (ESI), which went to effect on Dec 5th, 2021. ESI is one of the most commonly used pain management injections for seniors. About twenty-five percent of my patients have Medicare as their primary insurance and therefore are being affected by this new rule.

The new guideline requires that a patient has to have disabling pain for at least four weeks before an ESI can be done. Furthermore, a repeat ESI can only be done "when the first injection . . . (provided) at least 50% of sustained improvement in pain relief . . . for at least three months."

My patients who came to my office, writhing in pain, hoping to get treatment as soon as they could, were unanimously infuriated by these rules.

"Why don't these people, whoever came up with these crazy rules, try to live with this pain for even four days, not to mention four weeks, without treatment!" "I sometimes would need these injections every two months, sometimes every two years. My pain came back sooner than three months. It is not my own choice." They would say to me. Some patients with financial means would offer to pay cash to get the needed injection right away. Other patients, for Medicare patients are usually on fixed income and limited financial resources, would have to suffer and wait to get treated. How fair is this? How did our medical care system come to this point?

The above is guidelines for Medicare. Each insurance company has its own rules. It becomes impossible to keep track of each insurance company's specific requirement.

For example, one insurance company argues that a patient has to have a pain score of six out of ten in order to qualify for an ESI, forgetting the fact that a six out of ten pain can mean drastically different things to different patients. A number of six does not prove any meaningful clinical condition for patients.

We have to spend much longer to explain to patients why they cannot have treatments done right away. We also have to spend extra effort to document in patients' charts all these different timelines and measurements.

Our office staff has to call each insurance company to obtain the pre-approval. This process can take days to complete. Sometimes, each phone call a staff makes can take an hour because they have to navigate complicated phone systems and put on hold, in order to speak to a representative at the insurance company. Often, the insurance company requires their doctor to speak to me to further verify information before the pre-approval would be granted. All of these takes time. Patients are waiting. Patient do not want any delay, because they are in pain.

How can I pacify frustrated and angry patients, while I can hardly contain my own discontent?

"Nowadays, we doctors cannot decide what to do for you, we have to follow some books and rules set up by somebody else, who has never seen and evaluated you," I would say to my patients. The loss of autonomy and the added stress of documentation, and more documentation, have become increasingly prevalent in recent years.

One day, if I have to leave medicine earlier than I like, it would be because I am sick of dealing with insurance company rules and regulations. I am tired of having to ask for permissions (pre-approval) for everything I do for my patients, such as medications, injections, physical therapies . . . everything!

Why don't doctors hire more people to help with documentations and regulatory work? That would free up doctors' time to have real patient care. It all sounds reasonable. In reality, doctors would be under even more stress to increase productivity and workload, because the cost of running the office would escalate with more hired staff. It is a Catch 22, a vicious cycle. Who would not be burned out in this kind of environment?

My professor at a Harvard teaching hospital said to me, "The only way to reduce physician burn out is to reduce work, or not work as a physician at all. There is no way around it."

It turns out that doctors are doing exactly that.

The article "Fighting a Silent Epidemic" writes that, "In a recent joint study by the Mayo Clinic, the AMA and Stanford University, nearly 1 in 5 doctors say they intend to reduce their clinical hours over the next year, while 1 in 50 plan to leave medicine within the next two years. If even a third of these doctors follow through on their intentions, the nation could lose a physician pool equivalent to the graduating classes of 19 medical schools.[39]

39   https://healthtrustpg.com/?s=Fighting+a+Silent+Epidemic&post_type=page%2Cpost&cat=&order=desc

According to estimates from Atrius Health, the largest independent physician-led healthcare organization in the Northeast, every time a doctor quits, the cost of recruiting and training his or her replacement can range from $500,000 to $1 million.

And, the Blue Ridge Academic Health Group estimates that burnout costs the nation around $150 billion a year in physician turnover, lost productivity from early retirements and medical errors."

Poor patient care, shortage of physicians, that's when the whole healthcare enterprise tends to collapse. Ultimately, it is the patients who would suffer. It is the entire health care cost that would increase.

While there is no simple solution to the problem of physician burn out, there are little things that could booster your doctor's day and keep him or her going. Be understanding and appreciative to your doctors' effort. Believe me, we are the ones who really would like to make you better, almost more than yourself. No doctor wants to see his or her patients returning sick or unhappy. We all try our best. It helps when you tell us that you know that too.

"In any moment of decision, the best thing you can do is the right thing, the next best thing you can do is the wrong thing, and the worst thing you can do is nothing." — Theodore Roosevelt

Mayhem in Myanmar

Everyone has his or her own way to de-stress and recharge. My favorite choice is to go explore a corner of the world. When I am transported into a new place, I immerse myself into the local culture, people, and food. In places like these, I'm free from my daily stress and responsibility as a physician.

One January, my husband and I took a trip to the Far East and fell in love with the complexities and beauty of Myanmar. Myanmar, formerly known as Burma, is a Southeast Asian nation of more than a hundred ethnic groups, bordering India, Bangladesh, China, Laos, and Thailand.

One of Myanmar's main attractions is Bagan. Once the capital of a powerful ancient kingdom, Bagan occupies an impressive twenty-six square mile area. Standing on the eastern banks of the Ayeyarwady River, it's known for more than two thousand Buddhist monuments towering over the green plains.

One afternoon, we decided to make time to see the famous sunset in Bagan. Most of the two thousand Buddhist monuments are small stupas—small statuaries. They were scattered among the larger monuments. Some large ones had steps leading to a small platform where people could sit to watch the sunset.

Myanmar, at the time, had been through lengthy civil wars and multiple natural disasters. The country had poor infrastructures. Bagan, even though being the most visited place by foreigners, still remained a small city with developing facilities. One of the best stupas for watching the sunset was a few miles away from the paved road. We rented two bicycles and pedaled along the dirt roads connecting various stupas. We found and climbed up to the platform of the stupa. Comfortably ensconced among a few others, we awaited the magical moment as the sun drifted toward the horizon.

Suddenly, I heard somebody running in our direction, shouting, "Is there a doctor here? Is anyone a doctor?"

Oh, no. Being a doctor outside of our normal setting, such as a hospital and a medical office, is not the most desirable situation because it is out of our support system. I looked around, desperately hoped that somebody would respond before I did. The twenty or so tourists on the platform all looked at each other in silence. Before the man ran to a stop, I raised my hand, realizing that nobody else would.

He tried to catch his breath, then continued to yell, "Run doctor, run! There's a man in trouble. He is dying!"

I ran and thought to myself, "He's probably just being dramatic. Nobody should be dying. It is a sultry hot day in Bagan. Somebody probably fainted because of the heat."

"The doctor is here! The doctor is here!" The man ran in front of me was still yelling, toward a group of people congregated on the platform on a stupa next to ours. The crowd peeled open a narrow passageway for me. On the ground was a huge Caucasian man, well over three hundred pounds, lying motionless.

His face! I had never seen such a color on any human being's face. It was a deep but bright blue. In the operating room, I had seen patients with dangerously low oxygen levels. I had seen faces of patients near death. I had pronounced death for patients in the past. Their faces would look ashen, blue but with gray or purple coloration.

This blue reminded me of the blue color on a Pepsi Cola bottle label, utterly ominous on a human face. It shocked me back to reality. "Dammit! He is dying, or probably is already dead." My heart started to race.

I immediately sank to the ground to check his ABC's—his airway, breathing, and circulation. He had no pulse. His airway was unimpeded but there was no breathing. It was my turn to shout.

"He needs CPR right away! Call an ambulance!"

I immediately started doing chest compressions. "Push hard, push fast," I said to myself in my head to keep myself calm. "Place your hands, one on top of the other, in the middle of the chest. Use your body weight to help you administer compressions that are at least two inches deep and delivered at a rate of at least one hundred compressions per minute."

I have been involved in a good share of resuscitations—known as Code Blue in hospitals. As an anesthesiologist, my job was always at the head of the patient. I would place the breathing tube down the throat of the patient when needed. The nurses would have all the equipment and medications prepared, waiting for my orders. Chest compressions are always taken care of by other doctors or nurses. Everything would be done swiftly but in an orderly manner.

Now, I had to handle the chest compressions, and this resuscitation, without any equipment, medication, or other professional support staff.

Administering compressions to a three-hundred-pound man was not easy, especially by a person who wasn't even one hundred pounds. In fact, by the time I counted to thirty, my arms felt tired. I quickly realized that I would not last too much longer and the compressions would no longer be done effectively.

"Does anyone know how to do CPR?" I shouted, as I continued the compressions, and searched the group of people circled around us. They all looked stunned and nobody volunteered.

Sweat dripped from my face and neck. My heart raced with adrenaline. My arms became more fatigued and weak. I looked at the man's deep blue and motionless face, thinking to myself in despair, "He is going to die. He is going to die! Right here, right now!"

Suddenly, my husband appeared. "Do you need help?"

When he saw that I did not return right away, he decided to run over to check on me.

"Hurry, come over here to do CPR." He rushed over to join me and I quickly showed him—a man who had never had any medical training—how to do chest compressions.

As my husband took over CPR, I was able to have a chance to take charge of the person's breathing. My hands were badly trembling both from fatigue and the surge of adrenaline.

I quickly surveyed the patient again: still no breathing or pulse.

Then I tilted his head, lifted his chin, and stimulated his jaws: still no breathing. As I was getting ready to give him a rescue breath, a large woman came out of nowhere, stepped forward, and pushed me away, crying, "Don't touch him. You are hurting him. My husband is healthy. He is going to wake up. There's nothing wrong with him."

I was momentarily thrown into stupefaction and confusion. "Did I miss something? What am I doing here? Am I hurting him?"

The crowd pulled that woman back. I checked the vital signs once more. No pulse, no breathing.

"Stay away," I shouted. "He's going to die if you don't let me try."

I immediately felt terribly sorry for her. She and her husband traveled over half of the globe to Bagan for vacation. Now she might return home a widow. How tragic.

During this whole time, my husband never stopped his steady and strong chest compressions. I never appreciated his muscles more than that moment. Time was running out. I needed to give this man immediate rescue breaths. I kneeled at the head of the man again, my left hand tilting his chin, right hand pinched his nose closed, while keeping his mouth open. His mouth and tongue looked enormous. My mind was screaming, "How am I going to keep a good seal on this enormous opening with my small mouth? And here I am, about to put my mouth on another man's mouth, right in front of my husband." I felt guilty for having such selfish thoughts and yelled at myself, "Hurry! Hurry! He is going to die. Give him a good breath. Just try your best."

I took a deep breath and I was about to put my mouth on his, when all of a sudden, I saw a very slight movement in his throat. It was so slight, I thought I had imagined it. Did he just take a breath? I could not believe it. I stopped and watched him. He took another breath.

Then, another one. His breaths were shallow and irregular, but definitely there. Then, I saw something else I had never seen before. One pink spot, the size of a pin head appeared on his forehead as if a single distant sun shone on a deep blue ocean at twilight. Then, a few other pink pin head sized spots came out on his forehead. Slowly, these spots connected together to become blotches. I watched as pink blotches appeared on his forehead, cheeks and continued to spread across his face.

"Is this what we learned in medical textbooks identified as the 'mottled skin coloration'?" I thought to myself in awe.

Once his entire face became pink, I checked his neck and found a faint pulse in the carotid artery. We stopped chest compressions and waited as I monitored him to make sure he had a pulse and continued to breathe.

I didn't know what to expect. Unlike the movies and novels where patients magically recover to their usual health after doctors' heroic resuscitations, the reality is much grimmer. The majority of patients never make it. Even if patients live after resuscitation, they often are left with serious problems and need immediate hospitalizations. We wanted to check his blood pressure, EKG, get other lab tests done right away to prevent things going south once again.

"Where is the ambulance? Did anyone call for an ambulance?" I wiped away the sweat that dripped all over my face and finally had time to ask.

"Yes, I called the hospital to send an ambulance right away when he collapsed, before you arrived," somebody answered.

She, as I later found out, was the local guide for this group of tourists from Germany. She then proceeded to tell me that this man had climbed up about forty steps to the platform to watch sunset. When he reached the top of the staircase, he slowly collapsed, in silence.

As he lay on the ground turning blue, people realized it was not just a simple fainting spell and ran to look for help. I wasn't sure how long the entire process of our resuscitation lasted. It was probably less than ten to fifteen minutes, but to me, it was an eternity.

I sat on the ground, exhausted, but I still did not dare to let my guard down. Only the sight of an ambulance would allow me to relax a little bit. The description I received from the tour guide suggested that the man probably had some kind of heart-related event from the exertion of climbing up the staircase.

I anxiously searched the horizon of the great green plains for any sight of an ambulance but saw none. The man was taking regular and strong breathes. Slowly, he opened his eyes. He looked confused, still unable to move or talk, yet, I was relieved. He was alive.

Shortly thereafter, to my astonishment, he sat up with help. Although he was still in a daze, I never expected he would be able to do even that after what had just happened to him.

His wife hugged him and cried with joy.

"You almost died. This doctor here saved your life." A woman pointed to me.

He turned his head very slowly toward me, struggled a little bit, but couldn't make any sound. It felt good to see a little smile on his face. I was not sure how much he could comprehend at that moment. I was also uncertain how much I had done to save his life either. I felt that I was about to lose him multiple times. Yet, miracles seemed to happen every time I feared the worst.

As we were surrounded by thousands of Buddhist stupas, on this sacred ground, that had been worshiped by the masses for hundreds of years, some mysterious force was probably helping us all along.

When I made certain that the German man looked stable enough, I wrote down what I thought had happened and what I did along with my phone number on a piece of paper for them to give to the ambulance staff and their own doctor when they return to Germany. "Your husband is not healthy. He needs to go to a doctor right away." I made sure the wife understood what happened was not a trivial event.

My husband and I went back to the stupa where we had been. There was a small crowd there already occupying all the "good spots." But a number of people made room for us and let us sit in our original place.

"Doctor, you left your cell phone here. It is right there on the step. What you did was amazing," A tourist said to me. Others looked at me, smiling and nodding. The sky just turned vibrantly colorful and the sun was just about to set. We did not have to miss any of the beauty of the setting sun that day.

When we left the stupa after the sunset, the man looked practically normal. The German tour group was still waiting for the ambulance, which was called almost two hours prior. We decided together that it would be better for the tour bus to drive him to the hospital instead of waiting. He was able to sit on the staircase and moved down the steps on his buttocks with assistance. He waved goodbye to me and his face held a full smile.

For the rest of the trip, my husband was euphoric. He couldn't believe that he had taken part in such a dramatic event and acted as a good Samaritan.

I, on the other hand, had a complicated mixture of feelings. I was beyond ecstatic that the patient not only lived but looked very well. However, I kept flashing back to the event and tried to examine every single thing that I did.

Did I really access him correctly? Did he really have no pulse or was it just too faint for me to feel it? Should I have done more for his airway first, if he, in fact, had a pulse?

Instead of being an escape from stress from my work, the trip became a constant repeat of medical fact checking and critical thinking process. I couldn't sleep well as I lived with the "what ifs?" I continued to think of what would have happened if I had to watch him die in such a helpless situation. I had no equipment to intubate him, no intravenous access, no medications. His wife already thought that I was hurting her husband. What would happen if he had died? Would she blame me?

"You are too hard on yourself," my husband said. "If you were not there, he probably would have died because everyone else was too stunned to do anything."

He was probably right, but I still could not stop this seemingly endless self-criticism, because I wanted to learn from the incident. I wanted to be sure I could do the right thing the next time, should there be one.

After the trip, I had recounted the incident to some friends and colleagues. All my non-medical friends would "ooh and aah" in excitement and regard it as an amazing experience.

On the other hand, almost every single doctor friend remarked how fortunate I was. First of all, the patient was lucky to pull through and seem remarkably stable. With equal importance, I did not get myself in trouble.

"Imagine if this had happened on American soil: How much paperwork would need to be filled out?" one colleague said. "You could have been sued if the patient had died or lived with a bad outcome."

Really? Doctors can get into legal trouble, even if they act as good Samaritans? Would I have been blamed for my lack of ability to bring him back? What kind of legal responsibility do doctors have in a situation like this?

The term "Good Samaritan" is derived from a New Testament parable in which a Samaritan was the only passer-by to stop and render assistance to a man who had been left half-dead by thieves.

All fifty states and the District of Columbia have Good Samaritan laws. Each state law is different, but all states try to encourage healthcare professionals to help out in emergencies by restricting the liability of those who provide it. Unfortunately, doctors are not immune from liability when acting as Good Samaritans.

Protections offered by Good Samaritan laws require help to have been given during a true medical emergency. However, the term is somewhat ambiguous and different from state to state.

For example, cited in Gilman and Bedigian's article titled "Good Samaritan Laws," in New York, a physician returned to his apartment building after work. The wife of the building's manager stopped and frantically asked the doctor to help her husband who was sick. The doctor accessed the husband and called an ambulance. Her husband later died at the hospital. The wife ended up suing the doctor. The court ruled that no gross negligence occurred and that the assistance was offered during an emergency. The Good Samaritan law protected the doctor in this case.

A doctor in Indiana, on the other hand, was not so fortunate. The doctor was asked to go to a neighbor's house to check on her chest pain. After examination, he diagnosed the neighbor with pleurisy and prescribed medications. The neighbor went into cardiac arrest and died hours later. A lawsuit was brought against the doctor and the court found that the Good Samaritan law in the state did not protect the doctor.

When doctors try to help others as Good Samaritans, not only they put themselves at risk of legal trouble, they can put their own health and even lives at risk.

In Detroit, Michigan, on March 17, 2017, Cynthia Ray, M.D., a Henry Ford Medical Group pulmonologist stopped to help passengers trapped in an overturned jeep along Interstate 96. She was hit by a car herself in the process and passed away few days later.

One article on the Louisiana State University Law school website cited that it is a "pervasive myth of liability in the medical professions that physicians will be sued for a poor outcome if they stop to help a stranger in need." [40]

Gilman and Bedigian points out, "as long as the good Samaritan provided assistance in an emergency setting; the emergency setting was not caused by the volunteer, and the volunteer's actions were not negligent or reckless in nature; the volunteer should be protected from civil liability should an injury occur." [41]

Many sources also indicated that doctors almost never lost lawsuits if they acted as Good Samaritans.

However, having a good chance to win a law suit is hardly comforting, no matter how good this chance is. It is the fact that people still would initiate lawsuits against helping hands that is disheartening to the health professionals. When we try to help out in emergency situations out of kindness, in some cases, risking our own wellbeing, we can still get sued. Furthermore, even if these lawsuits' outcome was favorable to doctors, it would undoubtedly be emotionally and physically draining to deal with the legal process, let alone the work productivity and wage loss a doctor can suffer because of that.

---

40   https://www.law.lsu.edu/
41   https://www.gilmanbedigian.com/good-samaritan-laws/

If doctors can get in trouble helping people as good Samaritans, are doctors required to act in an emergency situation?

Does the doctor have to volunteer? No, nobody has to volunteer. In her article named "Liability risks for the Good Samaritan", Lee Johnson, JD states: "Many misguided people think Good Samaritan laws mandate that physicians volunteer to render aid in an emergency. They believe doctors have a 'duty to rescue,' but no such duty exists. Declining to volunteer is not a crime. There is no civil liability for not volunteering."

I believe that most, if not all of us, in or outside of the health profession, would like to do our part to help out in any emergencies, even there is no civil liability to do so. We, however, would like to do so without reservation. We would like the public to encourage everyone to volunteer by being understanding and less litigious. Imagine if people stopped to think about if they will be sued prior to offering potentially life-saving assistance. Valuable seconds, even minutes, could be lost.

So, next time, when someone is calling for help in an emergency, looking for a doctor, what will I do? I would still look around, hoping for another medical professional to be there, to work with me as a team. I would still raise my hand and do my best, even if I know the situation might not always be pretty. I believe in karma. If I would like somebody to volunteer to help me or my loved one in need one day if we should need it, then I need to do the same for everyone else. More importantly, as a physician, it is just part of the Hippocratic Oath that I took.

"If you could kick the person in the pants responsible for most of your trouble, you wouldn't sit for a month." — Theodore Roosevelt

Acknowledgement: A Double-Edged Sword

ONE THURSDAY, I was running around seeing patients as usual. My office manager ran down the hallway, holding something in her hand. "Look! Dr. Shue, look." She was holding the newest issue of the county magazine: "Look! Dr. Shue, you are on the cover of the magazine."

Our county is one of the biggest counties in the state. It has a very popular and nicely put together monthly magazine. Every year, it has an issue featuring the best doctors in their own specialties in the area. Doctors supposedly are voted by their peers-other doctors-to ensure the credibility of the list. I've never really understood how the selection process works. However, since I was among the "best pain management physicians" for a few times, I would like to think the process must be valid.

About three months before, the magazine had sent a photographer to take a few pictures of me working in the office to go with a little paragraph about what I do in this coming issue. They never told me that I would be placed on the magazine cover.

What a nice surprise. I am a cover girl. I never had thought that I would have this kind of glamour. Nobody did. When I showed her the magazine, my eight-year-old daughter asked me, "Mommy, how did you get to be on the cover of the magazine? How much did you pay them? One thousand dollars?" A patient saw the magazine in the waiting room and asked my staff, "Did Dr. Shue print this magazine? Is it a real magazine?" Another patient looked at me then pointed to the magazine and said, "Dr. Shue, you really look like this person on the cover."

The magazine organized a cocktail party for the six hundred plus doctors named in the "best doctor" issue. I wanted nothing to do with it. Not that I would not enjoy a glass of drink talking to my colleagues, it was because chances were, I would not even recognize who was who at a huge party like this. My ability of putting faces with names seems to be born deficient. I still remember that one time I was at a medical conference when a tall young man called my name. I desperately searched my memory but could not figure out who he was for the life of me. Then I found out he was one of my fellow physicians in the pain management department at the hospital.

Although we didn't see each other frequently, there were only six members in the department and I was the chief of the department who coordinated call schedules and meetings on a regular basis with every member. I was horrified. I managed to squeeze some painful smile on my face and said, "Wow, you look so dapper and different in street clothes, out of your usual scrubs. No wonder I could not recognize you."

My manager registered me for the cocktail party as soon as she found out that I did not plan to go. She would not take any excuses. I agreed with her: they put me on the cover of the magazine. They had done plenty enough to get me there.

To my relief, the cocktail party was much less painful than I had feared. People wore nametags. There was an enlarged 54x30 inch print of the cover-my picture-on display at the party, guarded by a staff from the magazine. At the end of the party, I asked him, "Hey, are you guys going to throw away that picture in the trash after tonight's event?"

"Yes, I am afraid so."

"Can I take it?"

"Sure."

That was how my big smiley picture got on the wall of my office waiting room instead of ending up in the garbage can. Now all my patients could see the picture and most had something to say about it.

Patients with savvy social skills would say, "Wow, Dr Shue, this is a great picture of you. You look so professional and smart in it." Most patients would say, "Dr. Shue, you look kind of different in the picture." Finally, a patient with brutal honesty said, "Dr. Shue, how did you get to look like this. You look nothing like this in real life." I laughed out loud and explained, "There is something called makeup. And there is another thing called Photoshop. That was how I get to look like this." Since I am too lazy to doll up every morning and it is impossible to photoshop my own face, I will have to keep disappointing my patients with my original mundane look.

At the cocktail party, a staff from the magazine said proudly, "The best doctor issue is our most popular issue of the year. Our subscribers are all over the county. People are going to keep this magazine and use it as a reference when they need to find doctors. They will be calling you." Sure enough, the phones rang.

My office staff and I were excited to see patients coming in because of the magazine cover. Free advertisement! How perfect! Slowly, however, I realized that these were a special group of patients.

Most of them came seeking second opinion. They usually would come with a tall stack of medical records. When I asked what treatments they had tried before, some of them were surprised and offended. "Dr. Shue, all my records are here. Didn't you review all of them?" It was hard to explain to them that reviewing every page would take up most of the appointment time. Furthermore, when I reassured them that their own pain management doctors had been doing appropriate treatments, they looked at me with despair and disappointment.

One of my patients wrote me a letter after she came from afar for her appointment. "Dr. Shue, it was with great anticipation I came to see you. You were my last hope. Seeing you on the cover of the magazine and reading all of the recommendations, I was so confident you could help me. You could not even provide me with a hypothetical answer, even after I explained the results of the various tests I had. I left with NOTHING. I can't say 'thank you,' because you left me with nothing to be thankful for."

I sympathized with my patients. I could only imagine their pain and frustration. I wish I could tell them I had a magic wand. I wish the magazine cover had turned my brain into a smarter and brighter specimen. Unfortunately, I am still myself. My brain did not possess anything different before and after that Thursday when my picture showed up on the front cover of the magazine.

As a physician, I am acutely aware of my limitations. I know the danger of playing God. I am comfortable with telling my patients that I am unable to help them. I am not ashamed to tell them that I do not know why they have pain or what to do for them. However, with this group of patients, my limitations all of a sudden are magnified. I try my best but still do not enjoy being frequently reminded of my failure to deliver, or to meet expectations.

I started to dread seeing patients seeking me out after the magazine cover. Yet, they kept trickling in.

JEFFERY CAME TO my office one early afternoon. There was an emergency to deal with before I could see him. A regular patient who came for a routine follow-up exam, passed out in a consultation room while waiting to be seen. We had to call 911 to take her to the local hospital.

I had to closely monitor this patient, starting an IV and making sure she was stable while waiting for the ambulance to arrive.

As the team of EMS responders finally came and flooded into the hallway and waiting room, I was busy giving a detailed report to the team regarding the incident. Patients on my schedule that afternoon had to wait. They were all understanding and accommodating, except for Jeffery.

Before I finally had the time to see Jeffery, a staff member warned me that he had come up to the front desk a few times, complaining that he had waited too long for me, despite the explanation of the emergency situation and hectic scene of the roomful of EMS responders.

I went into the consultation room when my emergency patient left in the ambulance, and I immediately apologized to Jeffery about the delay.

"Well, Dr. Shue, I hope there will be no delay like this in the future. I came here because I saw you on the cover of the magazine. I did my extensive research on you and read about you on every single doctor rating website. Had you not been on the cover of the magazine, I would have walked out of here a long time ago."

Jeffery stared right into my eyes. Before I could tell him which part of his words I would take as my luck or misfortune, he went on to tell me about his own problem.

He had been suffering from low back and leg pain for the six months or so. His pain was from a mild to moderate herniated disc in his lumbar spine, confirmed by his MRI imaging study. His history of pain and physical exam all fit the diagnosis.

"I am such a healthy person, doctor. There is nothing wrong with me. This pain is my only problem. It's so bad that I can't live my life anymore. I have been sitting around in the house all day, almost every day."

I glanced at the form he filled out earlier. It said that he had high blood pressure, high cholesterol, and diabetes type II. He weighed over 370 pounds and was five foot six inches tall. This meant that he qualified for the morbid obesity category because he had a body mass index of 41. A normal body mass index is between18.5 to 24.9 for a male patient. I questioned him about these diagnoses on the form.

"But the medications I am taking make me perfectly healthy now," Jeffery answered with confidence.

"What medical problems run in your family, like your parents or siblings?" I asked.

"Everyone was healthy. My parents both died in their sixties. I was their only child, no siblings."

"What did your parents die from? What medical issues did they have before they passed away?" I inquired.

"Oh, they died from old age. They had no problems before they died," Jeffery answered with distraction written all over his face.

How could anyone in his forties, or, in fact at any age, call himself healthy with hypertension, diabetes, and morbid obesity? And nobody dies in his or her sixties with a diagnosis of old age. His parents must have had severe medical problems to pass away at such an early age. Yet, I sensed that this conversation would go nowhere.

I changed our topic back to the treatment options for Jeffery for his low back pain and sciatica and Jeffery interrupted me. "I have tried over the counter medication, physical therapy, but nothing has helped. Physical therapy was making it worse. I need something stronger and better. Can't you give me a shot and take away my pain?"

I fast tracked my explanation to steroid injections and explained to Jeffery that not every kind of injection would be suitable for him. We decided that a lumbar epidural steroid injection would be the most appropriate.

"In addition to injections, the most important thing you need to do for yourself is to take off some weight for the sake of your spine and joints. It would make you feel much better."

I try to get a lifestyle and weight loss lecture in as much as possible for all my patients, especially those who fail to exercise or are overweight.

"You've got to be kidding me. I can't even move anymore. How am I going to lose weight if I can't exercise? You have no idea what I go through."

The Pandora's Box was officially opened. To make his point, Jeffery went into great detail describing how his pain had affected his daily routine, from getting up in the morning to going to bed at night. We had already made the diagnosis, discussed, and determined the plan for his treatment. I was itching to see my next patient, who had been waiting for a long time as well, due to the emergency. Jeffery seemed to have become immersed in his own autobiography and could not stop talking.

"Jeffery, it's terrible that your pain has affected your life so much. Why don't you make an appointment for the treatment soon?" Finally, I had a chance to cut in.

"How do I make my next appointment so that I do not have to wait like today?" Jeffery demanded.

"Early morning appointments are the best," I said, trying to be accommodating. "I always come in and start on time in the morning. If you are the first patient of the day, then you don't have to worry about uncontrollable events like today. It only takes one complicated patient to delay our entire routine."

"No, morning is impossible. I can only come in the afternoon. Make sure you are on time when I come back next time." Jeffery walked out of the door and then turned back. "By the way, next time, if you have an emergency, please call me first so I don't come and wait so long."

I was stunned, and then almost amused by what he said. I wanted to remind him the definition of an "emergency." I wanted to explain to him that I wish I could magically control the sun, the moon, the stars, and the exact flow of my office schedule. Yet, I smiled and kept quiet. Sometimes, it is impossible for a person to hear anything but their own words.

Jeffery came back on a periodic basis and had three lumbar epidural steroid injections over the next few months. The procedures went well, but they only offered mild relief for Jeffery's pain. Despite me urging him to watch his weight, he gained another ten pounds.

"Now, what? What else can you do for me?" Jeffery was obviously very frustrated.

I explained to him what he had was nerve root irritation due to anatomical changes in his spine. It was not severe enough to need surgery, but it would often take time and patience for his pain to improve.

The steroid injections were mildly effective. We could repeat them in the future for severe pain, but we would need to give his body a break in the next few months. I told him we could focus on other conservative and adjunctive treatments at this point. He should again, pay attention to weight loss and lifestyle modification to optimize his treatment.

"I don't want to gain weight either, but I just can't exercise," Jeffrey protested.

"I understand it is hard to exercise with pain. What about making some small changes in your dietary intake? Sometimes, changes such as skipping that one soda a day can make a big difference over time. I can send you to a weight loss specialist if you like," I suggested.

"I don't smoke, drink, or do drugs. I don't even drink much soda. Food is my only enjoyment. I have to make myself happy when everything else is going downhill for me. Don't you agree? Otherwise, what's the fun of living? I don't want to see any weight loss specialist. I don't need anyone to tell me what to eat or what not to eat. I need to be happy with my own life."

I disagreed with Jeffrey, but I found it difficult to argue against his rationale. But I did get the chance to say, "Jeffrey, are you happy with your life now? This pain is wearing you down and keeping you from what you like to do every day. Your weight is contributing to your pain, not to mention your other health problems like your high blood pressure and diabetes. If you don't change your lifestyle and lose weight, your back, your other joints, and your general health will all get worse."

"No. You are right. I am definitely not happy with where I am now."

"Jeffery, if you are not happy with your current situation, then it's time for you to make changes."

I saw the light at the end of the tunnel and was anxious to hit a home run with my point.

"That is exactly what I did. My pain is making me very unhappy. That's exactly why I came to you. Aren't you a pain management doctor? There must be something you can do to make my pain better. My other doctors gave me pills to take and make my problems go away. Now my blood pressure and sugar numbers are perfect. Why can't you give me a pill or a shot to make my back problem go away?" Jeffery was getting more and more irritated.

How did the conversation make such an unexpected turn? I felt exhausted. I tried to explain to him that his hypertension and diabetes had not exactly gone away. I also tried to tell him that what we doctors do would consist of an exceedingly small part of his health and pain control plan.

"Ninety percent of how your pain and health will progress in the future is controlled by your own hands," I continued.

"But it is your job to make me better, now," Jeffery insisted.

I remained quiet. When he realized I had no more rabbits to pull out of my hat to make his pain immediately evaporate into the air, Jeffery got up from his chair and shook his head.

"This is ridiculous. It was with great anticipation I came to see you. You were my last hope. Hearing about all these good things about you, and reading all of the great online recommendations, I was so confident you could help me. Yet, you could not even provide me with any relief. A pain doctor cannot even take away my pain. What are you good for then? What a shame that you were even on the cover of the magazine. You can't do anything to help me."

Jeffery rose from his seat and stomped out of my office.

Jeffrey had more than four decades of accumulated stress on a human body, as a result of poor lifestyle choices and a variety of other factors. Yet, he expected that a doctor could magically take all the misery and problems away, just like that.

I watched Jeffery as he left and was neither sad nor disturbed. It is nearly impossible to help a patient if he is unwilling to take ownership of his health problems and work with his doctors.

I gathered my thoughts and moved on to my next patient. I opened the chart. Under the question "how did you hear about us," it answered: "from the recent magazine." Oh, no, I said to myself.

I took a deep breath, went into the room, and introduced myself to the new patient: "How are you? I am Dr. Shue. I am an interventional pain management doctor. No less. No more."

"To see it, is to believe it." — Irene Tracey, M.D.

Seeing Pain With an MRI

THE JUDGE WAS wearing a plain black robe and sat behind a raised desk, directly across the room from me. Behind the judge was the great seal of the authority, the flags of the United States, and the state of New York.

On the left side of the room was the jury box, in which six jurors sat quietly, waiting. The defendant, the insurance company, sat on the right side of the judge's bench; the plaintiff, my patient Nicole, her lawyer, and I sat on the left side.

This is just like the movies.

I looked around the wood-paneled room with the classically recognizable seating arrangements. Dozens of famous and infamous film characters in courtroom dramas came to mind.

I tried my best to calm down, but this was the first time I was asked to appear in court as an expert witness for one of my patients. Vicious arguments and shouting matches depicted in courtroom movies kept making their way to my brain, as I waited for the judge to start. I took a deep breath and asked myself: How did I get myself into this?

I was in court to speak for Nicole, who had been my patient for two years. She had a thriving practice as a psychotherapist, yet her career was put in jeopardy when her car was hit by another car running a red light, leaving Nicole with two painful herniated discs in her neck. The constant shooting pain radiated down both her arms and prevented Nicole from sitting for more than twenty minutes at a time. She was even unable to use computers to write her patient notes without taking frequent breaks.

I had been treating her with cervical epidural steroid injections which offered moderate relief for a few months at a time. Unfortunately, Nicole still had to cut back her hours because the pain and limitation of movement lingered, and it never completely resolved.

Nicole had several cervical MRI imaging studies done since the accident and all the studies revealed the problematic discs. She also had a test called Electromyography (EMG) which measured her muscle response and the electrical activity in her arms, in response to a nerve's stimulation of the muscle. EMG is usually used to help detect neuromuscular abnormalities. In

Nicole's case, the EMG showed that she had significant cervical spinal nerve damage, corresponding to the level of her cervical herniated discs.

To me, it appeared that Nicole had a very straightforward case of cervical disc herniation as a result of the car accident. However, the insurance company was not convinced that Nicole should be compensated for her suffering, or loss of work productivity. As a result, a lawsuit was initiated.

Nicole and her lawyer asked me to be the expert witness on her behalf.

"All you need to do is to explain to the judge and the jury what happened to Nicole's spine due to the accident, and how you have been treating her neck and arm pain since the injury."

Nicole's attorney tried hard to prepare me before the court appearance, saying, "It's your first time in court, but you've been a pain management doctor for many years, so just be yourself; be a doctor. Educate your audience."

The entire afternoon was set aside for my appearance, giving me plenty of time to talk to those who stared at me. I had brought my spinal assemblage along and I showed the judge and jury Nicole's MRI films, pointed out each structure on the spine model, demonstrating how each epidural treatment was done.

Then I presented the EMG results, my physical examination records, and Nicole's pain score chart. I tried to use simple language so that everyone could follow. I also made eye contact with each juror to engage their attention.

To my amusement and irritation, two out of the six jurors promptly dozed off a few minutes into my lecture. I raised my voice to interrupt their naps, but it did not help. I even attempted to wake them up by the heat of a burning stare, but it was futile.

Before I became too distracted, as I thought about how our great judicial system was not exactly being perfectly executed with jurors sleeping through the process, I pulled myself back to my professional stance and continued to educate the rest of the audience.

After my presentation, the lawyers from both sides took turns asking me questions. The lawyer representing the insurance company was mild-mannered. He walked over, smiled, and asked, "Dr. Shue, is pain subjective?"

"Yes," I answered.

"So, when the patient told you she was in great pain; as bad as ten out of ten on the pain scale, did you have any way to prove that?"

I knew what he was trying to do. I wanted to explain to everyone that no one would subject herself to treatment with a 3.5-inch needle sticking into her neck, next to the spinal cord, risking the potential of being paralyzed, again and again, if she did not have real pain.

"It's a yes or no question, Dr. Shue." The lawyer read my mind.

I had to answer, "No."

"Thank you, doctor. I have no more questions."

Nicole's lawyer gave me a pat on the back for my overall performance in court. I was encouraged with what I thought would be the outcome of the court hearing. It was a straightforward case, and I was confident that the results would be favorable.

Soon after, the verdict was out.

Nicole lost the case.

Apparently, the defendant obtained a picture posted on Nicole's social media, in which she was driving a jet ski on vacation.

"How can somebody in so much pain drive a jet ski? Her pain is obviously not as bad as she pretended," the defendant's lawyer argued and convinced the sleepy jurors that Nicole's pain could not be real.

Nicole cried and said, "My lawyer tried to tell them that the jet ski was at a very slow speed, and I went on that vacation right after I had a treatment by you, which temporarily lessened my pain, but they did not believe that my pain was real. They kept saying that pain scores were subjective. I wish there was a method that could scan my brain and produce an objective score that could convince them."

I could only imagine Nicole's pain and frustration. As a patient, it's difficult to accept that her suffering was overlooked, and she was considered to be malingerer. Her pain scores used in my office to measure her condition and progress of her treatment were viewed as invalid because it is based on opinion and subjective reporting. As a physician, I also wish there were a method that could produce an objective score to prove that she was in real pain.

A machine and an objective pain score would have helped physicians determine who really would need to take a break from work, take pain medication, and receive more treatments. Imagine how much work productivity the society could preserve? Think of how much better health care resources could be allocated? Consider the lack of disagreements I would have with my patients? Everyone would be on the same page.

Now that problem may be in the process of being solved. Brain imaging is a whole new way of unraveling the secrets of pain and suffering. New research, begun in London, England, virtually illuminates the patterns of the brain's neural activities corresponding to pain.

Author Nicola Twilley introduced this cutting-edge technology, and Dr. Irene Tracey in her article named "The Neuroscience of Pain," published on June 25th, 2018 in The New Yorker.

In the article, Ms. Twilley first showed us that the history of pain research is full of failed and barbarous attempts to measure pain.[42]

---

42   https://www.newyorker.com/magazine/2018/07/02/the-neuroscience-of-pain

Nineteenth-century French doctor, Marc Colombar would measure pain by evaluating the pitch and the rhythm of the cries of the suffering.

By the twentieth century, doctors at Cornell University used a heat-emitting instrument known as a "dolorimeter" to apply precise instruments to the forehead. By noting whenever a person perceived an increase or decrease in pain to the forehead, they arrived at a pain scale calibrated in increments of "dols."

In 2017, scientists at M.I.T. developed an algorithm called, DeepFaceLIFT, which attempts to predict pain scores based on facial expressions.

Currently, all pain scales we use are subjective. The one I use in my office asks a patient to determine his or her pain score from zero to ten, zero being no pain, ten being the worst pain one can imagine. Since everyone's imagination and experiences are different, a five out of ten pain can mean very different pain level or functional ability to an individual patient. My patients often are irritated and refuse to answer when I ask them to give me the pain score. Some cannot verbalize a number to represent their pain. Some flatly think it is a useless practice and do not wish to participate.

When pain scores are self-reported, the accuracy of these numbers becomes questionable and prone to stereotyping and bias. Ms. Twilley points out that:" The 2014 edition of the textbook *Nursing: A Concept-Based Approach to Learning* warned practitioners that Native Americans "may pick a sacred number when asked to rate pain," and that the validity of self-reports will likely be affected by the fact that Jewish people "believe that pain must be shared" and black people "believe suffering and pain are inevitable." A 2016 paper noted that black patients are significantly less likely than white patients to be prescribed medication for the same level of reported pain, and they receive smaller doses. A group of researchers from the University of Pennsylvania found that women are up to twenty-five per cent less likely than men to be given opioids for pain."

Doctors and scientists have been searching for a way to objectively measure patients' pain. This information can help us identify who is really in need of treatment and attention, and therefore better allocate medical and social resources.

Dr. Tracey, a physician who directs Oxford University's Nuffield Department of Clinical Neurosciences had been using a powerful special MRI to study human brain activities to identify which brain area would correspond to pain.

Dr. Tracey published "the cerebral signature of pain"—the distinctive patterns produced by a set of brain regions that would light up during a painful experience, in 2007.

Author Twilley writes in her article: "Pain is enormously important in law," Henry Greely, the director of the Center for Law and the Biosciences, at Stanford University, told me. "It's the subject of hundreds of thousands of legal disputes every year in the United States." Many are personal-injury cases; others involve Social Security and private-insurance disability.

Greely predicts that, once researchers have collected enough data and developed standardized protocols, neuroimaging will follow in the path of forensic DNA—a scientific breakthrough whose results were eventually considered robust enough to use as evidence in court. [43]

Nicole was not fortunate enough to have this neuroimaging technology available to help her fight her case. However, I sincerely hope that one day doctors can have more tools to obtain deeper insight into patients' pain objectively. When asked "Is pain subjective?" doctors can then answer, "Pain is both subjective and objective."

---

43   https://www.newyorker.com/magazine/2018/07/02/the-neuroscience-of-pain

Epilogue

DIANA, A LOVELY woman, in her seventies, suffered for almost twenty years with chronic pain of various types. She complained that things had worsened a year before when her husband's health started to fail. She attributed her increased pain to the responsibilities she incurred when she became her husband's sole caretaker.

Her daily dosage of oxycodone was 80mg. She came to me to help her decrease her pain medication, because she just did not feel quite right taking them. She anxiously twitched when I discussed a plan to taper her dose to 60mg per day, as recommended by the CDC guideline.

"I will cut back your medication, step by step and very gently," I assured her. "You may feel some discomfort for the first few days, but you will never go into withdrawal when I do it so gradually. You can always call me if you have problems."

I encouraged Diana and she listened to me. I decreased her medication to 75mg a day. The following month, it was decreased to 70mg a day. With the reduced amount of drugs that she consumed, her pain overall did not change, but her mind became less foggy. Her new brain power made her feel decades younger. She was ecstatic.

"I want to keep going down with my oxycodone," Diana said when she reached our goal of 60mg daily. "I want to see how much I can push myself. I don't want to be dependent on those pills anymore. I want to feel myself again."

Diana was highly motivated, and we worked together as a well-oiled team. When she had increased pain, she would try meditation, exercise, acetaminophen, and ibuprofen. Before we knew it, she was completely weaned off oxycodone.

"Diana, you are done! You graduated from my office. I am so proud of you." I could not tell who was more joyous about the result, Diana, or me.

Medicine is a field that evolves and advances at a dizzying speed. In the years that I have been in practice, I have witnessed several generations of technological improvement of some procedures that we routinely use. New medications always appear for me to learn about and administer.

The paradigm of pain medication use has shifted since the opioid crisis was recognized. This has challenged us on how we should interpret and implement the guidelines from the regulatory government agencies, and academic professional societies. At the same time, we need to take into account each patient's individual pain and needs.

These questions are not easy to answer. I learn as I go, both from continuing academic education and the case studies of my patients.

My patients, I have realized, are my best teachers. I learn from each of them in terms of how they present their pain and disease; and how each patient responds to different treatments. The experience I gain and the lessons I learn from each and every one, have accumulated over time and become an invaluable resource.

More importantly, my patients have taught me things that I would have never learned elsewhere. They remind me not to forget to appreciate the little things that I take for granted; how important health, family and friends are and how life needs to be lived fully each single day because of its unpredictability.

I am grateful to be in the profession of medicine. I can't imagine any other job that could have done more to stimulate my constant desire to learn and give back. It provokes deep thoughts and appreciation for life and gives me insight into the complexity of human nature.

I'm an Interventional Pain Management doctor, a challenging specialty. Do I like to see my patients cured? Of course. Can I take away all their pain? Rarely. Will I ever find this job too hard to do? Sometimes. Will I ever give up trying?

Never.

Dr. Sabrina Shue received her undergraduate degree and M.D. degree from University of North Carolina at Chapel Hill. She completed her residency training in Anesthesiology from Harvard Beth Israel Deaconess Medical Center. She then completed a Pain Management fellowship at St. Luke's Roosevelt Hospital, an affiliate of Columbia University. She is board certified in both Pain Management and Anesthesiology. Dr. Shue is the current Director of Department of Anesthesia at Meadowbrook Endoscopy Center. She served as a former Director of Pain Management at White Plains Hospital. She has been practicing pain management and anesthesia in Westchester County, New York since 2007.

Linda Spear is an author and former journalist for *The New York Times*, where she reported on evolving health and human interest. Before her debut as a novelist with the critically acclaimed, *I Know You by Heart*, she served as manager of corporate communications at Ciba-Geigy, now Novartis. Currently she writes books with doctors who want to inform the public about developing advances in their specific fields of medicine. Her recent novel of suspense and murder, *The Iceman Checks Out*, received praiseworthy reviews by several newspapers and magazines. When she's not writing, she facilitates four Writer's Workshops for those who are interested in pursuing a journalistic career or just enjoy writing short stories, a memoir or even a book.

www.ingramcontent.com/pod-product-compliance
Lightning Source LLC
Chambersburg PA
CBHW031933190326
41519CB00007B/509